Air Purifiers
EXPOSED

Everything You Need to Know to Create the Ultimate Home Environmental Defense

Julian A. Cox

Seize It Health Matters ::: Spanaway, Washington

Air Purifiers Exposed
Everything you need to know to create the ultimate home
environmental defense

Julian A. Cox
Copyright © 2015

Seize It Health Matters
1604 200th ST CT E
Spanaway WA 98387
seizeithealthmatters.com
Photos by Eleny Cox

ISBN 978-0-9895773-4-2

Julian Cox has "'hit it out of the ballpark"' with his latest work, Air Purifiers Exposed. As a result of his research into this issue, he has quite eloquently set forth a resplendent treatise on this industry, its lack of veracity in its advertisements, and the potential pernicious side effects of these devices. He shares much more healthful means through which one can realize clean/healthful air quality indoors. The insights in his book will prompt me to share its significant points with friends, acquaintances, and clients who use these machines. It is a privilege to have read this book – Julian does great work!

Dr. Glen Hepker
Author of A Glimpse of Heaven

Julian A. Cox's book shatters the myths surrounding purifying systems and their use in the home. The fallacies related to air pollutants, asthma, and respiratory disease are examined in the clear light of science, where the human body is championed as the most effective purifying system of all. In place of expensive and ineffective machines, Cox shows us how to purify our home and work environments in the most efficient, healthy, and cost-effective way. We learn that plants play a fundamental role in removing pollutants and purifying our air. Not only do we learn which plants are the most resourceful to our atmosphere, but how to maintain those plants to get the best out of them. This book tells you everything you need to know to create the ultimate purifying environment.

Dr. Michael Murphy

ACKNOWLEDGMENTS

I'm thankful for the grace of God to be able to put such a great work together in order to help positively influence the lives of many.

I would like to thank Watsons for the use of its facilities in order to procure nearly all of the plant photos, along with the free use of the details on how to properly care for the plants.

I am also very thankful for the time my beautiful wife Eleny Cox spent taking pictures, and for the time that Janis (an employee of Watsons) took in guiding my wife to the plants she needed to photograph.

I am also thankful for the derivative contributions of the brilliant works of these great men:
Greville Macdonald M.D.
Ben Clark Gile M.D.
James Adams M.A., M.D., F.R.F.P.S.

Julian A. Cox
March 2015

INTRODUCTION

The purpose of this book is to help you realize what real air purification is and how to obtain it at a fraction of the cost of the various units available on the market. I will not go as far as to say that these companies are out to deceive the consumer, but you should know that the products they market do not do what you think they are doing.

So what might that be?

The answer is purifying your air.

This book will open your eyes to the facts about purifiers. It will teach you about real air purification and how to obtain it for yourself and your family.

We will cover other things such as:

- ☐ How air purifiers stack up to the true and most powerful heavyweights of the industry that cannot be patented.
- ☐ Finding out why many of the claims related to air purifiers are quite misleading, why this matters, and what you can do about it.
- ☐ Learning the most powerful way to create a true environmental defensive perimeter in your home or office that will not only improve health for you and your loved ones or employees, but also make breathing a lot easier.

CHAPTER 1

THE ASTHMA PITCH

Perhaps one of the greatest reasons air purifiers are touted is for asthma relief. The statistics confirm that there is a strong market for these products. According to the Centers for Disease Control and Prevention:

- Number of noninstitutionalized adults who currently have asthma: 18.7 million
- Percent of noninstitutionalized adults who currently have asthma: 8.0%
- Number of children who currently have asthma: 6.8 million
- Percent of children who currently have asthma: 9.3%
- Number of visits to hospital outpatient departments with asthma as primary diagnosis: 1.3 million
- Number of visits to emergency departments with asthma as primary diagnosis: 1.8 million
- Number of discharges with asthma as first-listed diagnosis: 439,000
- Number of deaths: 3,630

Also according to the CDC, asthma triggers may include:

- Tobacco Smoke
- Dust Mites

- ☐ Outdoor Air Pollution
- ☐ Cockroach Allergen
- ☐ Pets
- ☐ Mold
- ☐ Smoke from burning wood or grass
- ☐ Infections from influenza, colds, respiratory syncytial virus.
- ☐ Sinus infections, allergies, acid reflux, and breathing in some chemicals.
- ☐ Strong emotions that can lead to hyperventilation
- ☐ Physical exercise
- ☐ Medicines
- ☐ Bad weather
- ☐ Breathing cold, dry air
- ☐ Foods
- ☐ Food Additives
- ☐ Fragrances

Preventive medications for asthma, according to the Mayo Clinic, reduce inflammation in airways – the inflammation that leads to symptoms. Quick-relief inhalers (called bronchodilators) can open swollen airways.

Long-term asthma medications keep asthma under control and reduce the likelihood of an asthma attack. Long-term medications include inhaled corticosteroids (such as Flovent, Pulmicort, and Aerobid), and Leukotriene modifiers (such as Singulair, Accolate, and Zyflo). Long-acting beta agonists, which are inhaled medications, open the airways – but they may also increase the risk of an asthma attack. Combination inhalers such as Advair and Symbicort combine a long-acting beta agonist with a corticosteroid.

Quick-relief medications include short-acting beta agonists, which are bronchodilators such as ProAir, Ventolin, and Xopenex. Some physicians will also prescribe oral or intravenous corticosteroids.

According to the Asthma and Allergy Foundation of America, natural treatments that may be helpful include:

- ☐ Acupuncture
- ☐ Biofeedback
- ☐ Chiropractic spinal manipulation
- ☐ Hypnosis
- ☐ Laser treatment
- ☐ Massage, relaxation techniques, art/music therapy, yoga

Other non-drug options for controlling or avoiding asthma attacks include avoiding cigarette smoke and common allergans, along with food additives and processed foods. Many asthma patients are also sensitive to nitrates/nitrites and sulfites. Regular exercise and supplements of Omega-3 and magnesium can be helpful, as can reducing dietary protein and dairy products.

The statistics on asthma sufferers are serious and sobering, and I do not make light of them by telling you that air purifiers that are touted to bring asthma relief are not what they are cracked up to be. First of all, it is important to consider the method of relief that these companies' claims are heavily based upon. In a nutshell, the air purifiers' claims for the level of provided asthma and allergy relief rely solely on the quality of the filters the machines contain. Competing brands of air purifiers on the market make claims such as:

- ☐ A specified volume of air can be filtered so many times during an hour.
- ☐ It contains a charcoal pre-filter.

- ☐ A filter change light is included to alert you to replace the filter.
- ☐ A True HEPA filter is included, able to capture 99.97 percent of pollutants.
- ☐ The amount of microns at which the filter can capture pollutants.
- ☐ There are several layers of filters.
- ☐ It contains an activated carbon filter.

Have you ever wondered why the fuss over these different filters and asked yourself if it really matters? Even if you haven't, consider that the main selling point is that the airborne pollutants are the greatest threat to your health. As long as you are convinced that such an air purifier is the ultimate line of defense and greatest medium for alleviating your condition, then you'll believe that good filtration is the essential means of catching and removing large quantities of pollutants from your air. The assumption is that the reduction of pollutants' ratio in the air equates to your air being purified and your conditions being alleviated. It has been proven that air purifiers provide alleviation by removing these – but that is the sole point, alleviation. But alleviation does not equal solving or even addressing the root problem. Pharmaceuticals are wonderful at alleviating all sorts of ailments, but has anyone ever fully recovered from some serious condition due to a drug? One thing an air purifier is really good at alleviating is your hard-earned money on an ongoing basis as you replace all those expensive filters.

Let's have a look at some of these advertised filters:

A True HEPA filter is one that has passed the industry standards and is able to capture harmful particles that are easily inspired into the body and fall along the 2 micron range. This is why manufacturers state that the HEPA filter is able to capture particles down to .3 microns and lower. Just a note, if your machine specs only mention a percentage or lack the True HEPA label you may want to look into a different machine.

The charcoal pre-filter helps reduce odors if it is an activated charcoal filter.

The carbon filter is useful for eliminating most of the harmful gases found in your home as well as odors. Some machines have several carbon filters.

The more filters the machine has, the less stress is placed on all of the filters behind it, which allows them to capture more and more particles as the air passes through the machine and back into your home.

Activated Carbon

I will go so far as to say that if I had an air purifier I would most certainly be sure that it had an activated carbon filter. This filter alone is actually doing you a greater service then the HEPA filter, considering it is at least addressing part of the root cause of your asthmatic condition. Even this type of filter, though, is not as great as it's hyped up to be, if you have a better understanding of how it works. If you listen to what these companies tell you, it would seem that all the toxic gases in your air are being filtered out – but that is certainly not the case. Before I break it down, let me let you in on a little misconception.

It just so happens that the words activated carbon and activated charcoal are synonymous. There is no real difference between the two; they are exactly the same thing.

What makes activated charcoal or carbon so special?

"Activated" means it is heated or otherwise treated to increase its adsorptive power. Its internal surface area ranges from 950 to 1150 square meters per gram in order for the adsorbed chemicals to be trapped. To understand this adsorption process, just think of a special type of fly paper that sucks flies into it as they get within a certain range – and they won't be going airborne again. Simply put, this is the same way that activated carbon interacts with certain gases, the types that are poisoning you in your home and office.

Here are some things you should know about those activated carbon filters attached to your purifier and how effective it will be at removing those gases in your home:

☐ The rate of air flow and whether it is consistent or intermittent
☐ The type, concentration and diversity of the contaminants in your air
☐ The average and maximum temperatures in your dwelling
☐ The upper and lower limits at which these gases would explode

In the case of the adsorption of chemicals on carbon, they are more easily attracted to the carbon when the molecules of the volatile gases are closer to the same diameter of the carbon it is passing over. According to carbtrol.com, compounds having a molecular weight over 50 and a boiling point greater than 50 degrees centigrade are good candidates for adsorption.

Let's take a look at some common gases found in your home and office and see how they stack up to being adsorbed by activated carbon. These figures are available online at carbtrol.com – a manufacturer of equipment for pollution control and wastewater treatment that was founded in 1983.

- ☐ Tetrachloroethylene has a molecular weight of 165, boiling point of 121 degrees Celsius and capacity to be adsorbed by carbon of 35 percent.
- ☐ Xylene has a molecular weight of 106, boiling point of 138 degrees Celsius and a capacity to be adsorbed by carbon of 21 percent.
- ☐ Toluene has a molecular weight of 92, boiling point of 111 degrees Celsius and a capacity to be adsorbed by carbon of 20 percent.
- ☐ Benzene has a molecular weight of 78, boiling point of 80 degrees Celsius and a capacity to be adsorbed by carbon of 12 percent.

Just because the specs of some purifier or the market hype claims that all the gases will be removed from your air just because you have an activated carbon filter doesn't make it so. As you can see above that is far from being the case. Don't get me wrong, any percentage of harmful gases removed from your environment is significant. My aim is to empower you with the right knowledge so that you can be a purification expert and make the wisest decision for your wallet, yourself, your workers and family.

I will equip you with the information you need and give you suggestions on how and where to start. Keep in mind that even if air is not actively blowing through an activated carbon filter, it will still pull in any gases within its vicinity. What that means is that, with a little ingenuity, you have another cost-effective way aside from the purchase of an air purifier to remove these toxins from the air. You must understand that a HEPA filter is not able to capture those harmful gases in your air. The reason is simple: they fall in the 0.1 micron range and lower –a HEPA filter can at best capture down to 0.3 and some machines can capture down to 0.2 microns. This still is not enough to have an effect on the gases in the air. The focus on filters just doesn't amount to the significance that advertisers claim. Neither these filters nor the machines are capable of rooting out the real cause behind your asthmatic conditions, even though they may be able to remove air pollutants that further exacerbate your condition.

The Ultimate Filter

Did you realize that you are already in possession of the most state-of-the-art mechanism of air filtration known to man? You were born with it; it's your nose! It is truthfully your most powerful form of biological air filtration, and under normal circumstances it blows away all of the competition. Note my comment, "under normal circumstances," meaning that it has the ability, like any man-made filter, to become compromised. Compromise of your nose's filtration function can result from inhaling harmful substances, nasal injury or surgery, or because you don't breathe through your nose often enough.

While all of these are serious, the one most likely to affect you is the fact that you don't use your nose for the purpose it was created. Did you realize that your nose is actually the primary mechanism for respiration? "The nasal passages contain an exceedingly important, and the most intricate apparatus connected with the function of respiration, of the whole respiratory tract, and one whose normal functional activity depends on the integrity of the whole of the mucous membrane of the respiratory tract below."[1] This makes your nose the fulcrum upon which the state of your respiratory system balances.

Your ultimate filtration system not only filters the inspired air, but is also responsible for the supply of most of the moisture and heat of the inspired air. The function of your lungs is for the interchange of gases, and not the heating or moistening of them. Therefore it has been noted that nasal disease is apt to be associated with asthma in three ways:

- ☐ Reflexively, through the nervous system. The sensitive respiratory orifice is bound to send impulses to all parts of the respiratory tract.
- ☐ Where nasal disease is obstructive, the onus of warming, moistening and purifying the inspired air is thrown on the bronchi and lungs, which are thus being constantly irritated and made liable to more or less chronic inflammation.
- ☐ A diseased area is always a focus of inflammation, liable to attract disease to itself and to spread elsewhere.

These physiological and pathological considerations can't be emphasized enough, and are supported clinically and statistically. Clinically, by the fact that sneezing and

---

[1] Asthma and its radical treatment, James Adam, available on amazon.

then wheezing forms a routine sequence in many asthmatics. In many cases of asthma, nasal lesions are a common affliction. "This emphasizes the importance of nasal disease or defect as a factor in asthma and one that cannot be neglected in treatment," wrote Adam; "the basal factor is the toxemia, which is always present. Another way of stating the same thing is that asthmatics form a small minority of patients suffering from nasal disease."

Q: How often should one breathe through the nose to reap the most benefit and is there a certain method of nasal breathing that should be used?

A: You should breathe through your nose for both inhaling and exhaling as much as possible; there is no special method that is necessary for daily breathing, even if you have asthma.

Asthma is a disease that wreaks havoc on the respiratory system mainly through the inflammation of various parts of that system; it thereby causes a major inhibition of the airways. Whether you have asthma or not, it cannot be emphasized enough how integral is the functioning of your nose and its proper use in the protection of your respiratory system. Two of the most dangerous elements to your respiratory system are cold and dry air, as they are a very serious threat to the smooth mucosal lining of the entire respiratory tract, hence the inflammation that ensues with an abundance of cold and dry air through the mouth. Both are easily prevented by proper inspiration through the nose.

In a study that measured the breathing of chronic asthmatic patients during and after an attack of asthma, it was realized how great the difference was between the method of breathing as via nose or mouth. In the conclusion of the study, the authors noted that asthmatics may have an increased tendency to switch to oral breathing, a factor that may contribute to the pathogenesis of their asthma.[2]

Allergic Rhinitis and Asthma

According to several other researchers, allergic rhinitis, rhinosinusitis, and asthma frequently coexist in the same patients. Rhinitis is an inflammation of the nasal passages that makes nasal breathing difficult for an individual. The prevalence of allergic rhinitis among patients with asthma can be as high as 90 percent, and chances of an individual with asthma having an allergic type of rhinitis can be as high as 80 percent. This illustrates how integral the functioning of the nose is in the case of asthma. It also helps emphasize the importance of the use of the nose for the asthmatic.

Let's examine a few nasal facts:

The nose is your first filterable line of defense and the only orifice for filtration that you possess. Some of the solid particles passing through it are caught by the vibrissae, which are the hairs within the vestibule, and others get entangled by the mucus that lines its walls.

---

[2] www.ncbi.nlm.nih.gov/pubmed/10593789

Regardless of the atmospheric temperature as air passes through the nose, it is raised almost exactly to match the temperature of your blood before reaching the pharynx.

No matter how dry the external air is as it passes through your nose, it will be entirely saturated with moisture.

There are gaseous exchanges that take place within your nose between gases that are in the blood and that in the inspired air, just as it does within your lungs.

A normal functioning nose is free of things such as adenoids, sinusitis, polyps, and spurs.

Along with that a normal functioning nose is one in which the thin bone known as the turbinal does not touch the thin layer of cartilage known as the septum and allows the free passage of air. It is also one that inhibits the continuous transmission of impulses from an overly sensitive nose to the bronchial tree. "It is almost impossible to cure an asthmatic mouth breather," Adam wrote, "for cold, foul, un-moistened air perpetuates bronchial irritation." Mouth breathing creates somewhat of a chain reaction that begins with the interference of the oxidation of bodily tissues leading to a larger buildup of waste matter in the intestines. Oxygen is the fire that burns up the wastes as well as nourishes the cells and muscles so they can function properly. It keeps the bacterial equilibrium in check. Mouth breathing not only brings in less oxygen but also makes you more prone to stress because mouth breathing stimulates the sympathetic nervous system. The reduction in the oxidation of your body results in a greater abundance of toxins in the blood and leads to problems with digestion, which in turn has a direct impact on your nose. Adam summed up nasal disease and asthma in this way. "Toxemia alters the asthmatic so that his condition becomes like a powder magazine; nasal disease is apt to supply sparks which cause the explosions of asthma."

Is the picture becoming clearer to you now?

No matter the number of microns the HEPA/Charcoal filtration system is rated for, it does a wonderful job at removing pollutants – including bacteria, pollen, mold, pet dander, cigarette smoke, fumes, gaseous chemicals, and mold spores. The problem is that it fails to affect the temperature or moisture of the air that you breathe. Even your nose does a very good job of filtering out large airborne particles between the vibrissae and the mucosal lining. The fact that the purifier can filter out so many microns is not a good enough reason to purchase an air purifier. Even if it is listed as a medical device, it still fails to medically impact the true cause behind your nasal compromise.

How you breathe is the primary determining factor of whether you will suffer with respiratory issues – not the number or level of pollutants present in the air that you breathe. There are, however, certain pollutants (gasses) that do have a direct impact on your respiratory system regardless of how you breathe. While even the nose fails at their removal, the purifiers don't measure up all that well either. Proper breathing through your nose can help you avoid many of the pitfalls of respiratory failure, especially asthma. If you do have asthma, breathing through your nose can help alleviate some of your discomforts if you make it a habitual, lifelong practice.

CHAPTER 2

THE DUST HYPE

Along with the air purifier manufacturers' pitch of alleviating the pangs of the asthmatic is their defamation of the lowly dust mite.

☐ Is the dust mite really the scourge that these companies would have us believe?
☐ Does an air purifier truly prove its worth against them?

Dust Mites

They are likely the most vilified pollutant of the air purification industry. It is not that hard to see why – when you see magnified photos of them they resemble some creature from a horror flick.

But dust mites are not a threat to you or your pets, at least not in the sense that you must worry about being bitten or catching some contagious disease. They only eat dead skin.

Dust mites are microscopic little critters that live on primarily dead skin from both people and animals – skin that you and your pets are continuously shedding.

Their preferred places of residence are warm and moist places – or even better, a bed where you are snugly wrapped in your blankets.

Their feces and the skin they molt do pose a problem to certain individuals with allergic and asthma conditions, considering that that skin and feces make up a large part of the dust bunnies and airborne dust in your home.

The protein substances in the dust mite feces produce antibodies in humans who are allergic when these are inhaled or touch the skin. These antibodies cause the release of histamines, which causes nasal congestion, swelling, and irritation of the upper respiratory passages.

Things to keep in mind:

Dust mites serve a purpose; just like some birds of prey, they scavenge. They function as vacuum cleaners for your dead skin waste; the average individual loses about 10 grams of dead skin in a week. That number is even higher for your pets, so that means plenty of food for dust mites in your home.

The environment they live in is the determining factor for respiratory ailments – it's not the dust mites themselves.

You don't really have to be a clean freak to mitigate this problem.

Though it's true that the fecal matter and skin that dust mites produce can irritate your body, that does not make them the primary causal factor behind allergic and asthmatic conditions. It is easy to assume that if you focus on the dust mite itself – but it's really just part of a greater problem.

To illustrate, just consider the impact of intestinal bacteria on your body. It is well understood that bacteria are split into two basic groups – good and bad. The primary function of "bad" bacteria is the elimination of waste matter such as undigested food. These bacteria are quite fond of sugar, and you need the bad bacteria in your system just as much as you need the good bacteria. An excess of "bad" bacteria in the system, however, will lay the foundations for disease. Intestinal bacteria, like dust mites, provide a reasonable service for us, but they produce excrement that can cause us problems, but that excrement is not the real cause for the health issues that can result.

Manufacturers of air purifiers (and their ad agencies) emphasize that the skin and the fecal matter produced by dust mites is at the source of respiratory health issues. Negative health effects of mites, though, is determined by the amount of their food present in your home. If your home environment lacks fresh clean air – the windows are rarely if ever open – and you combine that with chemicals emitted from furniture, curtains, and carpets, and you often breathe through your mouth, then that environment seriously ups the effect that dust mites can have on your health.

Good ventilation is one of the most crucial pieces to keeping indoor pollutants in check. Some gases that directly affect your nose and respiratory system can become concentrated in a room when windows stay shut or are not open long enough. There's much more to it than just dust-mite-molted skin and fecal matter determining you air quality; it is the environment that influences the body – that's what affects your respiratory health.

On the other hand, it is the *mental* environment that directly impacts the state of the home environment. For instance, your knowledge and understanding of the household toxins you harbor and the reasons for their use will also set the stage for some of the ailments that beset you. Therefore, the less you are concerned about what you use to keep your home fresh and clean, the more concerned you will likely be about your growing health condition and the resultant medical bills.

The Dust

Airborne dust particles can be roughly grouped into two classes – first, the larger particles that are readily visible indoors or outdoors, and second, the smaller particles that are usually only seen when strongly illuminated. The coarser particles of dust, such as those swept into our faces on city streets in dry and windy weather, consist largely of small fragments of sand, broken fibers of plants, pollen, fine hairs, and the pulverized excreta of various domestic animals. They can also include ashes, fibers of clothing and other fabrics, particles of lime, plaster or soot, parts of seeds of plants, and various kinds of micro-organisms. The finer dust particles, which we may become aware of by the choking sensation they cause when inhaled (even though we do not see them), are most plainly visible as the so-called motes in the sunbeam that stream into darkened places. These are very light and consist of fragments of fine vegetable or animal fibers (such as cotton, wool, or other light materials), and of the greatest variety of microorganisms, either singly or in masses, such as bacteria and mold spores. These micro-organisms can also be found clinging singly or in clusters to the larger or smaller inorganic particles that make up the bulk of dust. Dry air, dry-ground surfaces, and winds favor the distribution of the fine particles that we call dust, and still air and moist ground tend to hold it in check.

If you consider the presence of dust particles in closed rooms, you'll see at once that the great renovating and cleansing agent that is so efficient outdoors is, except on special occasions, absent – this is the combination of winds, strong air currents, and rain. Once in a closed room, dust is very apt to stay there, unless some means is employed to get rid of it. Although the dust remains in the room, those heavier parts of it, which contain most of the bacteria, gradually sink to the lowest available levels: floors, shelves, and furniture. Therefore, the still air of a room may be almost completely free itself from micro-organisms (except for some of the lighter mold spores), within one or two hours. Of course, some currents of air (caused by a fan or by just walking about) will interfere with the complete subsidence of the bacteria-laden dust particles.

If you consider the constant tendency of dust particles to settle in quiet places out of strong air currents, and the fact that even ordinarily efficient systems of ventilation do not carry off any considerable portion of the dust particles from closed still rooms, you will conclude that ordinary living rooms, even though they are well ventilated, are actually dust and bacteria repositories. Furthermore, consider that a system of forced ventilation will cause large volumes of dust-laden air from outdoors to pass through, so we are actually, so far as micro-organisms are concerned, cleansing the air and sending it back out with fewer germs than when it entered – the germs settled slowly as the air made its way from the entrance to the exit of the ventilation openings.

Experiments have shown that allowing open air to blow through a room results in sweeping away a large number of the suspended micro-organisms in the air. However, this is not so for micro-organisms that already have settled on woolen or other fabrics, carpets, or upholstery that was already strewn with bacteria-laden dust.

Dust and dust mites are not in themselves a problem. The real issue is the environment and breathing correctly through the nose. This illustrates another flaw in the filtration process of the air purifier, i.e. the elimination of bacteria and dust already settled onto fabrics, furniture, plants, carpets, curtains, and other surfaces. These filters only have an effect on what is in the air. So what about those particles that are inhaled through the nose and trapped in the mucus, or even those that are taken in through the mouth and line the throat?

Biological Safeguards Against Dust Inhalation

The average volume of air that a healthy adult takes in at each breath has been estimated at about a half liter (about 30 cubic inches). The solid particles that we breathe in with the air, either through the nose or mouth, do not come back out with the expired air, but are retained on the moist surfaces upon which the air impinges going in and coming out. These foreign particles floating in the inspired air are caught largely in the nose or mouth or upper throat, while a certain number pass down into the bronchial tubes and lungs. A large part of this foreign material may be discharged from the nose, where it is caught in the mucous and secreted when irritated. A considerable portion of the inhaled foreign material gets into the mouth, and is spat out or swallowed. The floating material that enters the windpipe and bronchial tubes lodges on their moist walls and encounters a most efficient arrangement for its expulsion. Completely lining the larger air-tubes like a mosaic are myriad tiny cells shaped something like narrow short clubs set on end side by side. Projecting from the free ends of these cells are a number of minute hairs, so the cell looks something like a short club with a beard growing from one end. The whole inner surface of these air-tubes is lined with these delicate hairs called cilia, which are constantly swinging their free ends back and forth, bending as they recover, and then with a quick snap forward they send any small object that lodges on them sweeping upward toward the mouth, away from the delicate and sensitive lungs.

The movement of these cilia is less vigorous when the body is quiet, as in sleep, but increases in speed and force when the body is active. Most mucus or phlegm is apt to come up into the throat. This is because the increasing vigor of the ciliary movement as one's activity increases will sweep up the accumulation formed during sleep.

There is another very curious arrangement in the air passages for the disposition of small foreign bodies that are breathed into the lungs. There are certain cells in the body, called phagocytes, that float in the blood or tissues and occasional show up in the bronchial tubes or in the tiny air chambers of the lungs. When these cells encounter a foreign particle or a fragment of worn-out tissue anywhere in the body, they pounce on it, wrap themselves around it, and either digest it or destroy it or carry it off to some safe place of deposit, either inside or outside the tissues. These scavenger cells are usually abundant in the air passages, where they often take up dust particles of one kind or another, which are swept up into the mouth.

Despite these safeguards against the entrance of foreign bodies into the lungs, a considerable number of dust particles of one kind or another do get in, and they can lodge upon of the lungs' walls beyond the ciliated cells. In the walls of the tiny air-chambers of the lungs (where the blood is separated from the inhaled air by only a film) an important and subtle process occurs. The purity and virtue of the blood depends on this process, in which the blood gives up the carbonic acid and water it has gathered in its journey around the system, and takes in fresh supplies of oxygen.

People who habitually work in dust-laden air are susceptible to pulmonary disease caused by the lodging in their lungs of foreign particles of one kind or another. Even though comparatively small amounts of foreign particles in the lungs is a negative impact on your health, the lungs do establish tolerance of foreign particles lodged in their tissues. Therefore there may be considerable accumulation of foreign material in the lungs without any appreciable interference with health. In fact, the lungs of nearly all adults who live with considerable smoke and dust in the air, in polluted cities or in manufacturing regions, instead of being a delicate spotless pink color, are dotted all over with spots, streaks, and patches of inhaled dust particles that the body has not been able to get rid of and has stowed permanently in the tissues to mitigate interference with the action of the lungs. Here it remains as long as life lasts. However successfully the lungs may stow it away, there is a curious provision against its distribution around the body. As the blood circulates through the lungs (as well as in every other part of the body), a small amount of its fluid part oozes out through the walls of the vessels into the minute clefts and crannies of the tissues where the cells lie, nourishing the cells.

This nutritive fluid, or lymph, is gradually collected into a series of irregular narrow vessels that open into larger and still larger trunks, until finally it is poured back into the blood. If this lymph were contaminated or polluted by any harmful or foreign material encountered in the tissues, it would carry it straight back into the blood, where it could cause dire results.

But fortunately the lungs, as well as several other important organs of the body, are provided with a series of very efficient filters through which the lymph has to pass in its transit toward the blood current. Several of these living filters, known as lymph-glands (little reddish-white bodies) are grouped deep in the chest at the root of the lungs, and are so effective that although the lungs may be crowded with inhaled and stored dust particles, that the lymph filters may finally become black from accumulation. Even so, dust particles rarely get through them and into the blood or other parts of the body.

Why then do air purifier ads make all these sinister allusions to the danger of dust, if most of it is caught before it gets into the lungs, and that which does get in is disposed of in such an efficient way? The body rids itself of a great deal of the inhaled inorganic dust that lodges in the nose, mouth, and air-tubes of the lungs, and the body efficiently disposes of that which is permanently stowed away in the lung tissues themselves.

When considering the harmful effects of dust, it's important to separate inorganic from germ ingredients. The inorganic elements of dust in large quantities in inhaled air can cause disease of the lungs by the persistent irritation they induce. But it is only under exceptional conditions, as with coal-miners, grinders, and other workers in confined places with particles in great numbers that this occurs. Very moderate amounts of dust particles in sensitive people can cause such a degree of irritation of the respiratory organs as either to deprive them of robust health or predispose them to diseases they might otherwise readily resist. There is a reasonable case for dust being a problem, but it is certainly not the scourge it is claimed to be, enough to require you to purchase an air purification system. Neither are the dust mites, for that matter.

Air filtration or purification, regardless of the coal pre-filter, the HEPA filters, and the lowest micron reduction, just pale in comparison with our own organic filtration and defense mechanisms. Consider which is the more effective: the purchase of an air purifier or taking better care of your bodily systems and defenses through proper breathing and simple measures such as opening up the windows?

CHAPTER 3

PURIFIED AIR

Perhaps one of the greatest misconceptions about an air purifier lies with the name itself. If you purchased an air purifier to actually purify your air, then you have surely been misled. The reason is simple: air purifiers are not designed to purify air, and it is impossible for them to do so. The problem lies with the misunderstanding of the difference between purified and filtered air. Consider what the manufacturers say degrades your air or makes it impure:

- ☐ Dust.
- ☐ Dust mites.
- ☐ Pollen.
- ☐ Cigarette smoke.
- ☐ Mold spores.
- ☐ Bacteria.
- ☐ Pet dander.
- ☐ Fumes.
- ☐ Gaseous chemicals.

While all the above certainly can make breathing difficult (depending on how much is present and the size of the room you are in and whether the windows are open or closed) you are still able to breathe just fine. The essential element is the ability to breathe *properly* as it relates to air purity.

Fresh air consists of 78 percent nitrogen, with 20.9 percent oxygen and 0.3 percent carbonic-acid gas.

You know which of the three humans depend upon the most: oxygen. The quality of oxygen present is the true litmus test for the purity of the air we breathe. Have you ever heard an air purifier company claim that their system actually increases or adds to the oxygen component in the air it supposedly purifies?

Fresh air consists of about 20.9 percent oxygen, and the volume of air in a single breath is about 20 cubic inches – just a little smaller than a baseball.

Adults take about 18 breaths per minute or 1,080 breaths in an hour, which is equivalent to breathing about 12 cubic feet of air. By the end of the day for most people, that is about 350 cubic feet – about the same size as a 7x7-foot small room.

Because of our oxygen needs, the loss of even 1 percent of the 20.9 percent of oxygen that fresh air contains makes air less supporting. The air you exhale has less oxygen than it did when you breathed it in. Less oxygen of any degree equals air degradation and impurity. When the air is degraded and you are present in it for long durations, besides the other pollutants in it, it can lead to eventual health issues. If you quit breathing, or you're breathing air that has already been breathed in and out (by you or others), then carbon will accumulate in the blood. In just half a minute, the blood in your arteries is noticeably darker; in 45 seconds it takes on dusky hue, and in 90 seconds the blood in your arteries becomes nearly black. If a room experiences a rise in carbonic acid in 5 percent of its volume, death can result.

Think about what happens when you rarely or never open your windows, and you have pollutants floating around, and you're breathing through your mouth instead of your nose. Let's say we run several competing brands of air purifiers in this room at the same time. Which of them is going to purify your air on top of removing all the contaminants? You might check off the boxes for pollen, cigarette smoke, and most gaseous chemicals, but the most important box goes left unchecked. None of the systems will add quality oxygen back into the air of that closed-up room.

What is an air purifier really purifying? The answer to that is a resounding **nothing**. Air purifiers do not purify the air. Then what are they actually doing? They are *filtering* your air. This is the only thing actually being accomplished besides fanning back out recycled filtered air. This is the sole reason that so much advertising emphasis is focused on the amount of microns and the quality of the filters that the systems have. If you were to remove the filters from the machines, then all they would do is suck in and spit back out the same air.

But the problem with these air filters is the notion that they are sold as "air purifiers," something that they completely fail at and are incapable of doing. Just removing the pollutants from the air doesn't purify the air. Neither do those pollutants present in the air really "degrade" the air or make it "impure." If it is truly the case that dander, mold spores, and dust actually create impure air, then what is the difference between outside air and indoor air? Think on that and consider that the same so-called impurities exist both indoors and outdoors. For that matter, how do you think they came to be indoors in the first place? That's right, they hitched onto your clothes, shoes, socks, and hair. If we believe what the air purification companies say is impure air, then all outside air is impure.

It's impossible for the air outside to become totally impure. Why? The reason is simple, outside air is being constantly rejuvenated with fresh oxygen. However, there is really a very obvious difference when you take into consideration the air in and around a metro area compared with the air in a mountain wilderness. On an elementary level, the fewer trees and plants present, the less oxygen there is produced. Also in the city, you must contend with the air pollution from vehicles and factories and CO2 emissions that will have a direct impact on the quality of oxygen available in the air. The other factor is the wind – the element that helps to keep things moving; it is the same basic difference as water in a stagnant pond and a flowing stream.

Let me briefly return to the subject of asthma. Much of the industry advertising focuses on pollutants as a great determining factor in the symptoms of the asthmatic. However, consider the difference between a person in a closed-up room and one who opens up their windows every day.

Outdoor exercise improves the metabolism of the asthmatic. Sitting in a warm and stuffy room will exacerbate problems; a quick bicycle ride or a brisk walk can alleviate them. The exercise and fresh air encourage active oxidation in the tissues and result in a freer airway in the nose.

The only way to really purify your air is to exchange stagnant oxygen-depleted air with fresh air rich in oxygen. It is nearly impossible to enjoy healthy oxygen-rich air if you run a filter spitting out recycled, degraded air while you stay inside with the windows closed day in and day out. This is a perfect recipe for causing or exacerbating respiratory issues, especially if you add habitual mouth breathing into the mix. Air filters, also, are not designed to deal with increasing carbonic acid gas levels in the air.

An Inside Job

If you are in a very small room with no source of incoming fresh air, your breathing will change the air in the room so much that if you stay there long enough, you will die. The Black Hole of Calcutta, according to Wikipedia, was a small dungeon in the old Fort William in Calcutta, India, where troops held British prisoners of war after the capture of the fort in June of 1756.

One of the prisoners, John Zephaniah Holwell, claimed that British and Anglo-Indian soldiers and civilians were held overnight in conditions so cramped that many died from suffocation, heat exhaustion, and crushing. He said that 123 of 146 prisoners died. His claims, though, have been controversial – a 1959 study by author Brijen Gupta suggests that the number of those in the Black Hole was about 64 and the number of survivors was 21.

Fortunately, air rarely gets that bad in any room. But in any room, impure air mixes with pure air and quickly degrades its quality. This degradation of indoor air quality can cause:

- ☐ headaches, fatigue, shortness of breath
- ☐ sinus congestion, coughing, sneezing
- ☐ eye, nose, throat, or skin irritations
- ☐ dizziness and nausea

In a room with closed windows there is a potential increase of CO_2 levels during the morning hours until outside temperature reaches a comfortable level and the windows are opened. While severe or even moderate health effects are not linked to the rise in CO_2, it will:

- ☐ induce drowsiness
- ☐ inhibit concentration

- ☐ impair cognitive function
- ☐ contribute to headaches

You can't assess the condition of the air by the looks of the room, because you can't see the air itself, and after you're in a room for 10 or 15 minutes, you don't notice the smell of the air in the room like you did when you first walked in – you will notice degradation of air quality in a room when you come in from outside.

A little experiment with ink and water will help illustrate this. Put about ten drops of ink into a glass of water, and it will mix together quite quickly. Put in fifty drops, and the water will be very black. In a similar way, "used" air from the lungs of about thirty children mixes with pure air in a schoolroom and degrades it for breathing.

How much fresh air is really necessary for us to breathe in? Consider a box that is one foot long, one foot tall, and one foot wide – a cubic foot. Recommendations for children's health include about 3,000 cubic feet of fresh air every hour. Adults need about 3,500 cubic feet of fresh air per hour or about 1 cubic foot of fresh air per second.

Active Ventilation Systems

Back in the 1970s during the international oil embargo, the U.S. made efforts to foster domestic energy independence. At the time, about one-fourth of the electric grid was used by commercial buildings. Various public agencies, state agencies, and school districts took measures to reduce this level, and one move was to decrease the volume of fresh air that came in through ventilation systems – along with shutting them down periodically.

What does this have do with you?

Since 1973 there have been standards for the volume of fresh air that is mixed in with a heating, ventilation, and air conditioning system. Originally the design was for a maximum of 15 cubic feet of fresh air per minute for every person in the building. This was prior to the oil embargo. Since the embargo, though, many systems were reduced to mixing a mere 5 cubic feet of fresh air per person. This isn't even close to adequate, especially if the ventilation system is the only means of providing fresh air. This change, and our heavy reliance on active ventilation systems, created a new ailment, sometimes called "sick building syndrome."

In Your Quarters

Whenever you come into a house from outside, pay attention to how the air smells. Notice it when you first go in, because you will get used to the air after you have been in it awhile, and then you cannot tell whether it has an odor to it. If it does, or if it does not seem as fresh and pleasant as the air outside, you can assume it is not pure. The levels of carbonic acid gas as measured by parts per 10,000 in the air is how we gauge whether the air is impure and unfit for breathing. This ranges lies between 2 parts and 12 parts per 10,000 – and the higher it gets the unhealthier it is. At levels exceeding 12 parts per 10,000 your senses become so dulled that you will no longer be able to smell the difference in the purity of the air; at lower levels the smell is more noticeable.

To show how little time it takes to change the air, suppose you shut all the windows of your room and light an incense stick. See how quickly the smoke floats around here and there. Soon the room is quite saturated with the fragrance. Now open the windows on opposite sides of the room and see what happens. If a breeze is blowing in from outside, you will find that it pours in at one window while the smoke streams out the other, and the room is cleared in almost no time. Of course, the impure air is pouring out of the room with the smoke, and the pure air is coming in just as fast.

Now pause for a moment and look around the room you are in and see whether you can tell how the fresh air gets in and how the old air gets out. You may have to judge by the windows. Notice which are shut and which are open, and see whether a breeze is blowing; then try to decide whether enough air comes in to supply all who need it. It's important to ensure, for at least part of the day, that windows on opposite sides of your home or office are open to create cross ventilation. There's no way to tell exactly how wide open windows need to be, or for how long, because it depends on the size of the room and the number of people in it, as well as the size of the windows and the direction of the prevailing air flow. When a breeze blows, an opening of an inch or two may be enough, but on a quiet day in summer the windows should be wide open. Some people think that the hallway door will provide all the air they need, yet they do not take pains to see that the hallway itself is actually receiving outdoor air.

By opening your windows all year round, at least for a bit each day, regardless of the weather, you allow the wind to stir things up and move contaminants around and out. It will not have a significant effect on pollutants that have already settled on your curtains, clothing, carpet, and other surfaces. Neither will an air purifier, for that matter

Another method that is touted to purify the air is beeswax candles. Even if you are burning a beeswax-based candle, you are not purifying the air any more than a machine is, considering that neither of these methods does anything for the fresh exchange of oxygen. Beeswax does neutralize the positive ions brought forth by the very things that an air purifier sucks up, but it does not produce any fresh oxygen in the environment, so what is it really purifying? You already know the answer: it is just filtering the air on a molecular scale without recycling it. Either way the same degraded air remains, just as it does with the machine.

CHAPTER 4

NATURE'S WAY

So how can you achieve purified air? It will probably not come as a surprise to you when I say: PLANTS. It is impossible to achieve air purification without them, considering they are the *only* natural oxygen-producing factories that exist upon the face of the earth. There really is no other sustainable, cost-effective, easier, or better method of purifying your air than nature's way.

Plants eliminate carbonic acid gas, which they actually rely on for their existence; and they produce a fresh supply of oxygen. Plants cause both a removal of carbonic acid gas and a fresh exchange of oxygen. Does this not, in fact meet the criteria of air purification? Machines and beeswax cause neither, only the neutralization of pollutants. Plants, like all natural surroundings, also produce negative ions that help disrupt some of the electromagnetic effects of technology devices. An increase in negative ions in the air can also benefit your psychological state, health, and overall wellbeing.

The Scourge of Ozone

Another selling point of certain brands of air purifiers is their ability to reduce indoor ozone levels. This colorless gas is formed when oxygen reacts with other chemicals, and some of the side effects of overexposure include:

☐ Pulmonary edema

□ Hemorrhage
□ Inflammation
□ Disruption of proper lung functioning

Because many people in developed countries spend 80 to 90 percent of their time indoors, indoor air pollution has become a public health risk. According to *Science Daily*, the United Nations Development Program in 1998 estimated that more than 2 million people die each year because of the presence of toxic indoor air, while other studies estimate that 14 times as many deaths occur globally from poor indoor air quality compared with outdoor air pollution. The economic consequences of polluted indoor air are considerable; one Australian study estimated that the cost of unhealthy indoor air in that country exceeds $12 billion annually.

Cost-effective and easy-to-use methods are needed to eliminate or reduce ozone concentrations. Activated charcoal filters reduce air pollutants, but installation and maintenance costs can be high. Researchers have investigated alternatives – such as indoor plants to improve indoor air quality and health.

Ozone Generating Purifiers

Aside from this, it is important for you to realize that some of those air purifiers being sold on the market are actually responsible for raising ozone levels in your home to a degree that they could actually trigger smog alerts for outdoor air.

If ozone generators are ineffective at removing pollutants, and they indeed pose health risks to users, why are they still being sold? The unfortunate answer is that misleading advertising by manufacturers is very effective, and government agencies do not have the authority to fully regulate these devices.

According to the California Environmental Protection Agency, a device that produces ozone is rightfully labeled an ozone generator, but that ozone is often misleadingly labeled as activated oxygen, energized oxygen, or super-oxygenated air.

Manufacturers claim that the reactive nature of ozone can purify the air and remove airborne particles, chemicals, mold, viruses, bacteria, and odors. Ozone, however, does not clean the air except at extremely high, unsafe ozone levels – and even then it is only partially effective.

Ozone also does not remove particles (e.g. dust and pollen) from the air, including the particles responsible for most allergies. Research shows that ozone generated by air purifiers does very little to remove chemical pollutants. In fact, ozone reacts with chemicals in the air to create other pollutants, most notably formaldehyde and ultrafine particles.

Some consumers purchase air purifiers to eliminate odors, but ozone concentrations below health standards do not remove many odor-causing chemicals. Ozone also deadens one's sense of smell. Not only does this disguise odors, it can also have the risky effect of decreasing your ability to detect high levels of ozone.

Before you make a decision, let's have a look at some studies on ozone-generating purifiers. According to the Environmental Protection Agency (2007) here are some study results on these machines:

They produce indoor ozone levels several times the state outdoor health standard of 90 parts per billion (ppb) for one hour. They also exceed the 8-hour standard of 70 ppb.

In one of the tests conducted, a level of 300 ppb was measured in a house after 1 or 2 hours of ozone generator use. Indoor ozone levels were about twice the health standard when the generator was set on high, whether the central fan was on or off.

Ozone levels were almost twice the health standard in the room, even with the device at a medium setting. These concentrations are equal to or worse than a first-stage smog alert. The ozone concentrations produced by these devices can easily exceed health-protective standards.

If you study publications addressing ozone you will find no conclusions to dispute the evidence presented here about the dangers of ozone to your health. This is further echoed by the Air Resources Board (as cited by the Environmental Protection Agency in 2007), "We strongly advise against the use of ozone generators in occupied spaces. Other governmental agencies agree with this advice."

If you are concerned that your air purifier could be the cause of increasing ozone levels in your home, check the list at www.arb.ca.gov/research/indoor/o3g-list.htm online.

According to the Air Resources Board it is a *partial* list of air cleaners sold as "air purifiers" or ozone generators that can emit ozone. This list includes air cleaners sold primarily for residential use, plus some for commercial, in-vehicle, or personal use. Inclusion on the list was based on information available at the time.

NASA Research

In the later part of the 1980s there was a significant study conducted by NASA and the Associated Landscape Contractors of America (ALCA) that spanned the course of about two years. Researchers were interested in finding a way to create healthier and more breatheable environments in outer space. "They found that certain tropical plants, commonly used as houseplants, were quite effective in removing formaldehyde, benzene, and trichloroethylene from the air and replacing it with breathable oxygen," explains The Pros Who Know. Dr. Bill Wolverton was the head of one of the research teams with the task of studying houseplants in this manner. They tested the effect of 15 houseplants on three pollutants known to be present in spacecrafts: benzene, formaldehyde, and trichloroethylene, which are present in your home and probably your workplace.

So how do they end up there in the first place?

Benzene: common sources of benzene in your environment include:

- ☐ Inks.
- ☐ Oils.
- ☐ Paints.
- ☐ Plastics.
- ☐ Rubber.
- ☐ Dyes.
- ☐ Detergents.
- ☐ Gasoline.
- ☐ Pharmaceuticals.
- ☐ Tobacco smoke.
- ☐ Synthetic fibers.

Benzene can negatively affect your health by:

- ☐ Causing headaches.
- ☐ Causing dizziness.
- ☐ Causing drowsiness.

☐ Causing confusion.
☐ Loss of consciousness.

It is also a known carcinogen. All these are results of exposure in gaseous or chemical form at high levels. In your home your rate of exposure is higher if smoking occurs often and for homes with attached garages. Most exposure to benzene happens through inhalation.

Formaldehyde: common sources of this in your breatheable environment include:

☐ Foam insulation.
☐ Plywood.
☐ Pressed-wood products.
☐ Grocery bags.
☐ Waxed paper.
☐ Fire retardants.
☐ Adhesive binders in floor coverings.
☐ Cigarette smoke.
☐ Natural gas.

Formaldehyde can negatively affect your health with:

☐ Irritation of the eyes.
☐ Irritation of the throat.
☐ Irritation of the of the nasal cavity.
☐ Coughing.
☐ Chest pains.
☐ Bronchitis.

Of all the gases, formaldehyde has been found at very high levels in indoor air because of its use in many building materials, along with its broad use in daily consumer products. The highest levels are found in newly manufactured homes and mobile homes.

Trichloroethylene: Most common sources of trichloroethylene include:

☐ Metal degreasing.
☐ Dry cleaning industries.
☐ Printing inks.
☐ Paints.
☐ Paint removers/strippers.
☐ Lacquers.
☐ Varnishes.
☐ Adhesives.
☐ Typewriter correction fluids.
☐ Spot removers.
☐ Rug-cleaning fluids.

Trichloroethylene causes negative health effects including:

☐ Damaging your central nervous system.
☐ Causing dizziness.
☐ Causing headaches.
☐ Causing confusion.
☐ Causing euphoria.
☐ Causing weakness.
☐ Causing facial numbness and weakness.

Trichloroethylene can also cause harm to the immune system and endocrine system, as well as cause problems with development.

Trichloroethylene has also been associated with kidney, liver, and cervical cancers.

The good news is that although these chemicals can easily find their way into your home and work environment, in a controlled environment the NASA study found that specific houseplants were able to remove **at least 87 percent** of these irritants in just a 24-hour period. Plants by their nature purify the air and improve its quality. The tropical plants in this particular NASA study showed us something very significant:

Tropical plants grown as houseplants in cooler climates are effective at processing gases and chemicals. Because they naturally grow in dense rainforests with very little light, they are very efficient at photosynthesis – absorbing gases from the air. As they transpire or emit water from the foliage, air is drawn down around the roots, where root microbes consume the chemicals that are absorbed. Plants useful for reducing toxic chemicals indoors include common houseplants that you can find at your local garden center. Two of these very common plants include Gerbera Daisy and Pot Mum.

Through the process by which plants naturally sustain themselves from sunlight (photosynthesis), they also take in certain pollutants along with carbon dioxide. Plants have a natural way of removing pollutants, purifying your air, and even performing air filtration on a molecular level, through the negative ions they produce Nature's methods are far superior to any man-made machine – and houseplants are less expensive, more attractive, and more effective than any "air purifier" device.

These gases, commonly found in your home, can be harmful to visitors even if you don't have any respiratory illness or issues. What to do if you're expecting a guest with asthma? A very good first step would be ventilating the house for several minutes or an hour before the arrival of the guest, especially if you don't have an air filter – but it's an effective means of freshening your indoor air even with a filter. Likely offenders on the list of household products that commonly emit gases include:

- ☐ Synthetic candles – replace these with pure soy or beeswax-based candles.
- ☐ Newly installed carpeting or fairly new carpeting – use fresh-air ventilation, recommended houseplants and air filters in rooms with new carpet.
- ☐ People who smoke should ventilate the house well and then smoke only outdoors during the stay of a guest.
- ☐ Replacing common detergents and cleaners with products that are natural-based can be very beneficial.
- ☐ Replacing household cleaners such as window, floor, counter, and stovetop cleaners with natural-based versions is also a good start.
- ☐ Keeping products such as varnishes, lacquers, paint, paint remover/strippers, and cleaning fluids in a place that is less trafficked such as a garage will greatly reduce the breatheable concentration of gases that emit.

At the top of your list for a healthy home environment should be ventilating the rooms with fresh air and replacing household products with more eco-friendly formulations.

Another point you should understand about negative ions and the whole concept of molecular air filtration is that negative ions bind to pollutants and drag them down onto your floors, furniture, curtains, and other surfaces. But once they lose their charge, those same pollutants will be set free again. Household cleaning such as sweeping, mopping, and vacuuming furniture and floors is a necessary part of a routine to keep your environment clean.

While these were not part of the focus in the NASA study, there are other contaminants to consider in your home:

Xylene: Common sources of xylene include:

- ☐ Solvents.
- ☐ Coatings.
- ☐ Paints.
- ☐ Varnishes.
- ☐ Newly installed carpeting.
- ☐ Cigarette smoke.

Xylene can negatively affect your health in ways such as:

- ☐ Causing fatigue.
- ☐ Causing headaches.
- ☐ Causing drowsiness.
- ☐ Causing lack of coordination.
- ☐ Damaging the central nervous system.
- ☐ Irritating the respiratory system.
- ☐ Irritating the eyes.
- ☐ Irritating mucous membranes.

The main process by which you are exposed to xylene is inhalation. Xylene levels are generally much higher indoors than outdoors because of the products harboring this gas. The more of these products you have in the home, the higher its concentration in your environment.

Toluene: Common sources of toluene include:

- [ ] Adhesives.
- [ ] Inks.
- [ ] Nylon.
- [ ] Dyes.
- [ ] Cosmetic nail products.
- [ ] Synthetic fragrances.
- [ ] Cleaning agents.
- [ ] Paint and other coatings.

Toluene can negatively affect your health by:

- [ ] Causing fatigue.
- [ ] Causing sleepiness.
- [ ] Causing headaches.
- [ ] Causing nausea.
- [ ] Damaging the central nervous system.
- [ ] Irritating the upper respiratory tract.
- [ ] Irritating the eyes.
- [ ] Causing soreness of the throat.

Toluene concentrations indoors are typically higher than outdoors because of gases emitted from household products such as those listed above. Your workplace environment could have high toluene levels if people there frequently deal with printing or painting or activities using solvents.

Ammonia: typical sources of ammonia in your environment include:

- [ ] Carpeting.
- [ ] Photocopiers.

- ☐ Window cleaners.
- ☐ Floor waxes.
- ☐ Other cleaning products.

Ammonia has negative effects on your health that include:

- ☐ Causing rhinorrhea.
- ☐ Causing scratchy throat.
- ☐ Causing tightness in the chest.
- ☐ Inducing a cough.
- ☐ Causing dyspnea.
- ☐ Irritating the eyes.

Ammonia is a naturally occurring substance both in your body through cellular respiration and also in nature. Naturally occurring ammonia is regulated by natural processes, but it can build to toxic levels in your body. If you are overexposed to ammonia through the daily upkeep of your home or on the job, these are not natural occurrences that will work themselves out without potential risk to your health.

Formaldehyde, xylene, and toluene all have a direct impact on your nose and respiratory system. Of all the gases mentioned above, these three are most likely to be concentrated in your home just from building materials and household products.

Regardless of how well a carbon filter removes these gases from your air, it doesn't beat nature's own purification system – ventilation by wind power. The problem – and the challenge – is the environment you create in your home that threatens your health and that of the ones you love. The good news is that you can change it once you have the knowledge to implement that change.

The most cost-effective and simplest way to reduce the concentration of gases in the home or office is through ventilation, with windows open on opposite sides of the structure, as often as you can for as long as you can tolerate. The longer the windows are kept open, the better. Just remember besides reducing the gases inside, you also want to bring in fresh oxygen. Of course air purifiers don't hurt when you need to shut things up, but neither do plants that can do the same. Even better is when you combine the use of plants, ventilation, and air filtration. It is up to you and your budget, but if you proceed carefully you can get the most for less.

CHAPTER 5

THE PURIFYING POWER OF PLANTS

In this chapter you will learn about what plants are needed in order to neutralize the chemicals likely to be found in your home.

Plants for Benzene

Aloe (Aloe Vera) falls into a class of plants known as succulents, and the following care should be kept in mind for a healthy and useful plant.

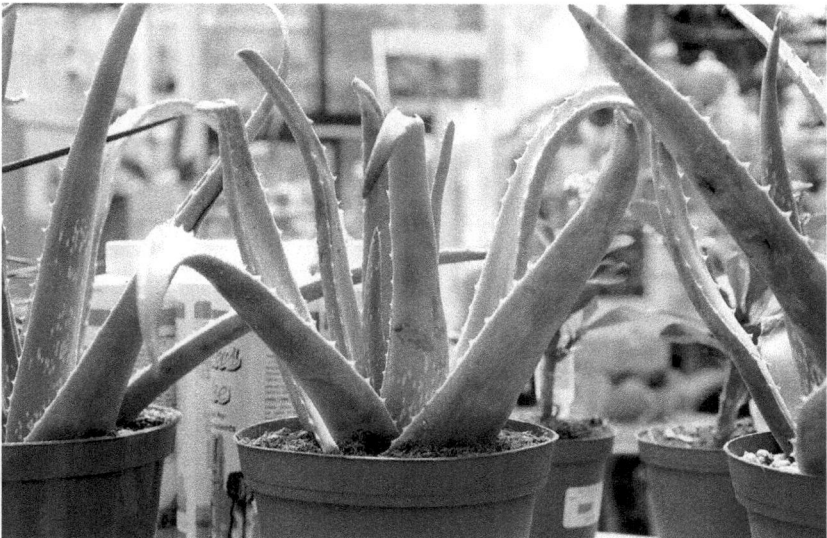

Light: Bright light is needed. A south-facing window is best, but if there is too much light the leaves will turn brown or white. If there is not enough light the stems will elongate and you will end up with widely spaced leaves.

Temperatures: Like most succulents, night temperatures between 50 and 55 degrees are preferred, with daytime temperatures between 70 and 85 degrees.

Water: Water aloe generously in the summer. Let it dry between watering and take care not to over-water it.

During the winter, watering should be cut back to about once every other month. Above all else, do not allow the plant to sit in water.

Signs of over-watering: The plant will become soft and discolored and the leaves could be yellow or white or could lose color.

Signs of under-watering: Aloe will stop growing during growing season (spring and summer) if it's needing water, and will begin shedding its leaves. Aside from its purification and filtration benefits, aloe also provides a natural medicinal gel within its leaves that can be used topically on cuts and burns or mixed into smoothies for a powerful health drink.

Spider Plant (Chlorophytum Comosum)

Light: Bright indirect light – but avoid direct sunlight.

Temperatures: You will do well to keep a spider plant between 60 and 75 degrees; don't keep it in an environment below 50 degrees.

Water: Just ensure the pot has good drainage. Don't be afraid to allow the soil to dry out between waterings.

Don't use a pot more than 2 inches bigger around and deeper than the pot you got it in.

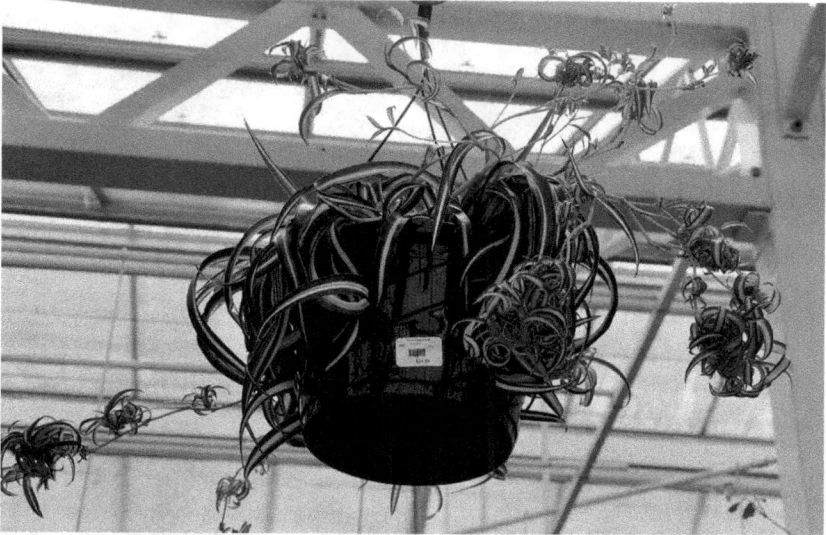

Weeping Fig (Ficus Jenjamina)

Light: bright light is necessary.

Temperature: Average warmth, minimum 55 degrees.

Water: Water with care and allow the soil to dry out to some extent between waterings. Use tepid water and apply very little during the winter months.

Humidity: Mist leaves occasionally in summer.

Repotting: Avoid frequent repotting. Repot in spring every 2 years until the plant is too large to handle.

Propagation: Get stem parts in summer if stems are non-woody. Use a rooting hormone and provide bottom heat (from a heating pad) if possible.

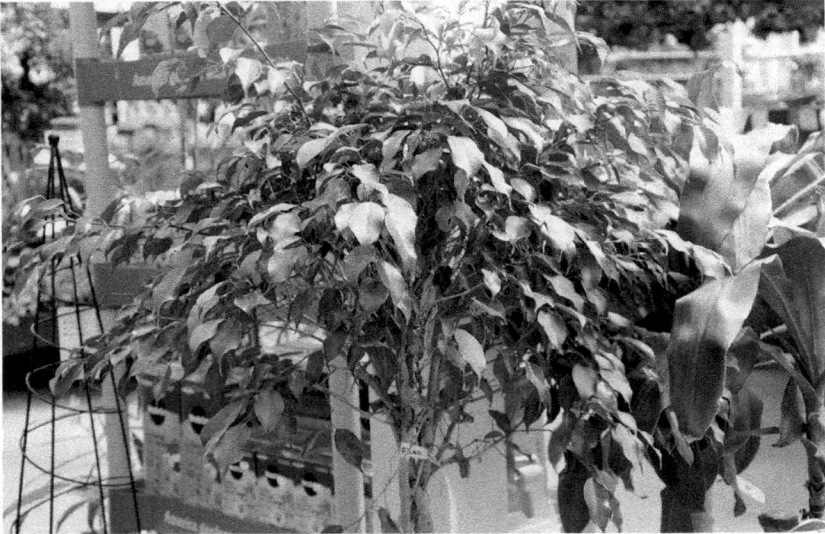

Gerbera Daisy (Gerbera Jamesonii)
Light: Bright indirect light – but avoid direct sunlight.
Temperatures: Keep between 60 and 75 degrees.
Water: Make sure the pot has good drainage. Don't be afraid to allow the soil to dry out between waterings.
Don't use a pot more than 2 inches bigger around and 2 inches deeper than the pot you purchased it in.

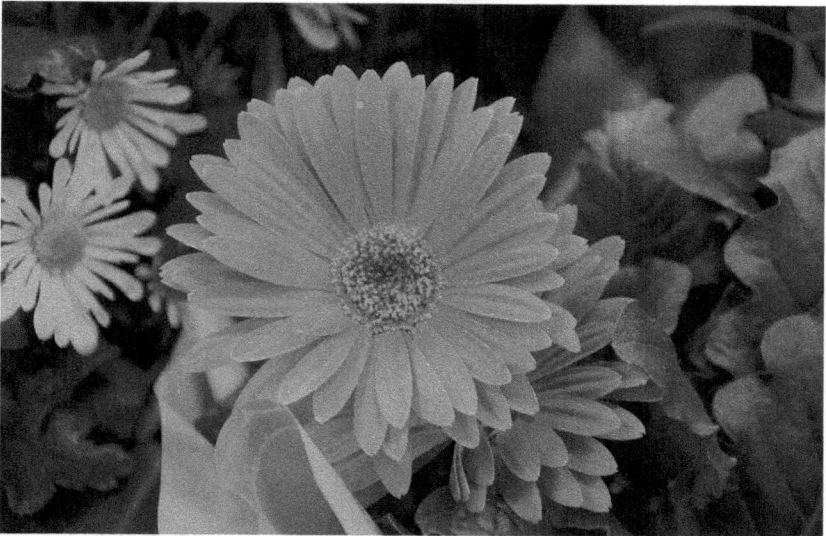

Peace Lily (Spathiphyllum)

Light: Semi-shade in summer and bright light in the winter.

Temperature: Warm or average warmth with a minimum of 55 degrees.

Water: Keep soil moist at all times, but reduce watering in the winter.

Humidity: Mist leaves very frequently.

Repotting: Repot in spring every year.

Propagation: Divide plants at repotting time.

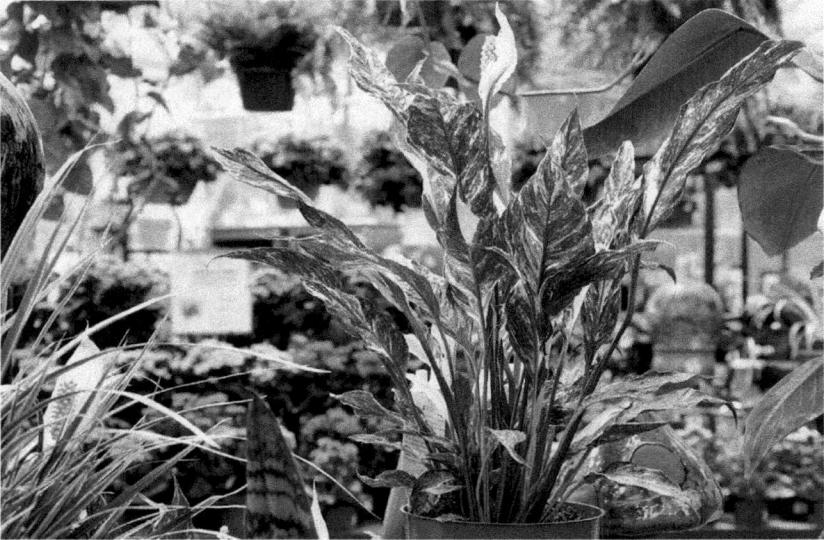

Janet Craig (Dracena Deremensis)

Light: Light shade is the best general condition, close to an east or west window if possible.

Temperature: Average warmth, minimum 55 degrees in winter.

Water: Keep the soil moist at all times. Reduce watering in the winter, but don't let it dry out.

Humidity: Mist leaves regularly.

Repotting: Repot in spring every 2 years.

Propagation: Remove crown from old leggy canes and plant in potting compost. Use a rooting hormone and provide bottom heat, or air layer the crown before potting. Two- to three-inch pieces of stem can be used as cane cuttings.

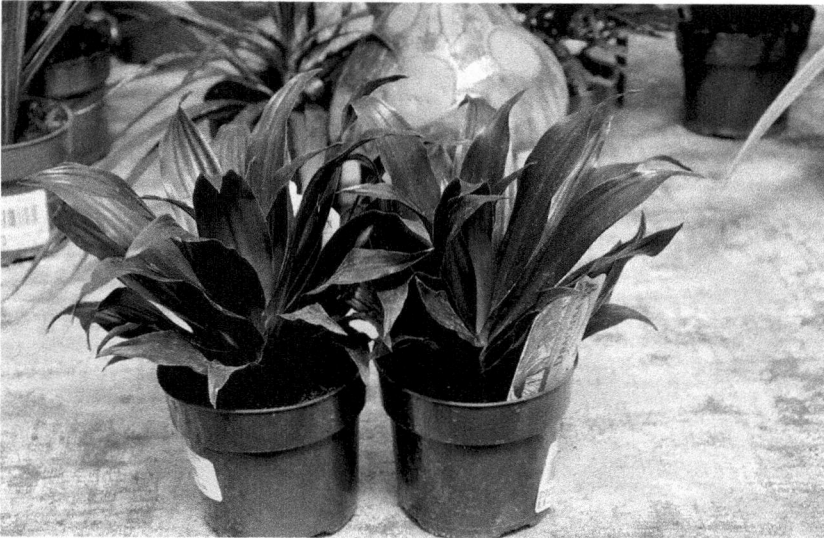

Special Problems: If you get leaves with brown tips and yellow edges, the common reason is dry air. Most Dracaenas need high humidity, so surround the pot with moist peat and mist it regularly. Cold drafts and under-watering can have a similar effect.

If you get leaves that are soft and curled with brown edges, then the temperature is too low. Dracaenas will quickly show these symptoms if kept close to a window on cold winter nights.

If you see lower leaves that are yellowing, and it occurs slowly, then this is probably just a natural sign of old age.

If you get leaves with brown spots, you are probably under-watering. The soil must be kept moist.

If you see leaves with bleached dry patches, move the plant to a shady spot because it is probably getting too much sun.

If your plant dies, it's most likely because of over-watering in the winter or air temperatures that are too cold.

Warneck Dracaena (Dracaena Meremensis 'Warneckii')

Light: Light shade is the best general location, close to an east or west window if possible.

Temperature: Average warmth, minimum 55 degrees in winter.

Water: Keep the soil moist at all times. Reduce watering in the winter but don't let it dry out.

Humidity: Mist leaves regularly.

Repotting: Repot in spring every 2 years.

Propagation: Remove crown from old leggy canes and plant in new potting compost. Use a rooting hormone and provide bottom heat. Two- to three-inch pieces of stem can be used as cane cuttings.

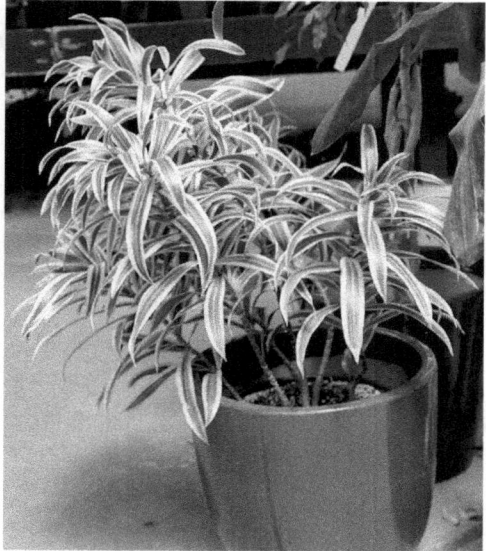

Special Problems:

If you get leaves with brown tips and yellow edges, the common reason is dry air. Most Dracaenas need high humidity, so surround the pot with moist peat and mist it regularly. Cold drafts and under-watering can have a similar effect.

If you get leaves that are soft and curled with brown edges, then the temperature is too low. Dracaenas will quickly show these symptoms if kept close to a window on cold winter nights.

If you see lower leaves that are yellowing, and it occurs slowly, then this is probably just a natural sign of old age.

If you get leaves with brown spots, you are probably under-watering. The soil must be kept moist.

If you see leaves with bleached dry patches, move the plant to a shady spot because it is probably getting too much sun.

If your plant dies, it's most likely because of over-watering in the winter or air temperatures that are too cold.

Red-edged Dracaena (Dracaena Marginata)

Light: Light shade is the best general location, close to an east or west window if possible. Unlike the other two dracaena, this one can grow in the shade.

Temperature: Average warmth, minimum 55 degrees in winter.

Water: Keep the soil moist at all times. Reduce watering in the winter, but don't let it dry out.

Humidity: Mist leaves regularly.

Repotting: Repot in spring every 2 years.

Propagation: Remove crown from old leggy canes and plant in potting compost.

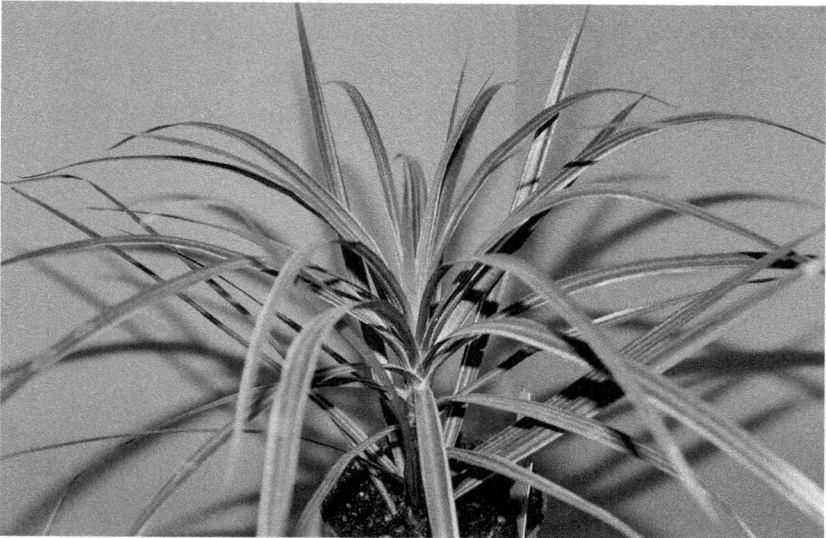

Use a rooting hormone and provide bottom heat, or air layer the crown before potting. Two- to three inch pieces of stem can be used as cane cuttings.

Special Problems:

If you get leaves with brown tips and yellow edges, the common reason is dry air. Most Dracaenas need high humidity, so surround the pot with moist peat and mist it regularly. Cold drafts and under-watering can have a similar effect.

If you get leaves that are soft and curled with brown edges, then the temperature is too low. Dracaenas will quickly show these symptoms if kept close to a window on cold winter nights.

If you see lower leaves that are yellowing, and it occurs slowly, then this is probably just a natural sign of old age.

If you get leaves with brown spots, you are probably under-watering. The soil must be kept moist.

If you see leaves with bleached dry patches, move the plant to a shady spot because it is probably getting too much sun.

If your plant dies, it's most likely because of over-watering in the winter or air temperatures that are too cold.

Bamboo Palm (Chamaedorena Sefritzii)

Light: Keep in partial shade.

Temperature: Average warmth, minimum of 50 degrees in the winter.

Water: The first need is for good drainage, because all palms detest stagnant water at the roots. During the winter, keep the soil slightly moist. Water more liberally in spring and summer.

Humidity: Mist leaves if room is heated. Make sure to occasionally sponge mature leaves. Try to avoid having drafts.

Repotting: Repot only when the plant is thoroughly pot-bound. Palms don't like disturbance. Compact the new compost around the soil ball.

Propagation: From seed. A temperature of 80 degrees is required, so propagation is difficult.

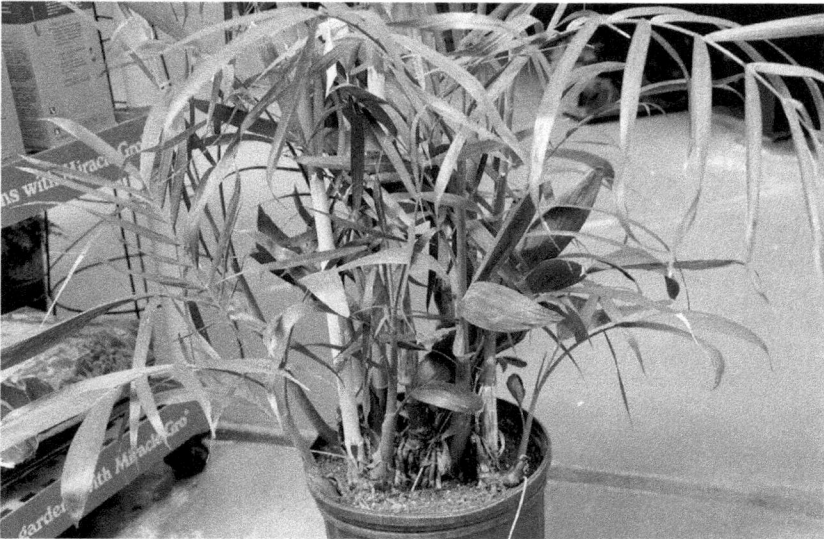

Special Problems:

If you have leaves with brown tips, this is most likely caused by dry air. Mist the plant regularly during hot weather. This can also be caused by under-watering, cold air, or damage from touching.

If you have leaves with brown spots,- it's often caused by leaf spot disease from overwatering or sudden chilling. Just remove the affected foliage and improve the growing conditions. Another cause could be the use of hard water.

If you have yellowing leaves, it's likely a sign of under-watering. You don't want the roots to dry out during the summer months.

If you have brown leaves and droop, this is natural for the lowest leaves. Just remove by cutting, but not by pulling. If the browning is accompanied by rotting, then the problem is most likely from overwatering.

Pot Mum or Florist's Chrysanthemum
(Chrysanthemum- orifolium)

Light: Bright indirect light, but avoid direct sunlight.

Temperatures: Keep it between 60 and 75 degrees.

Water: Just ensure the pot has good drainage. Don't be afraid to allow the soil to dry out between waterings.

Don't use a pot more than 2 inches bigger around and 2 inches deeper than the pot you purchased it in.

If you have pets, keep this plant out of their reach; it's toxic, especially to cats, dogs, and horses.

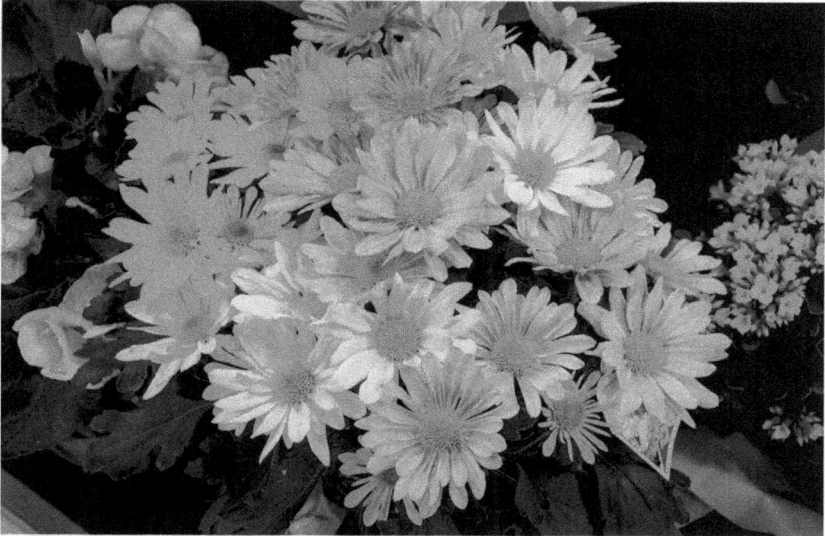

Plants for Formaldehyde

English Ivy (Hedera Helix)

Light: Keep out of direct sunlight. Keep in light shade or moderate brightness.

Temperature: Average warmth, minimum 55 degrees in winter.

Water: During winter keep the soil just moist, and make sure it is not waterlogged. For the rest of the year, water thoroughly and regularly.

Humidity: Keep the air moist in the summer and keep in a heated room in winter. Surround the pot with peat and mist the leaves.

Repotting: Transfer to a larger pot in spring every 2 – 3 years.

Propagation: Cuttings require warm conditions.

This plant is toxic to cats.

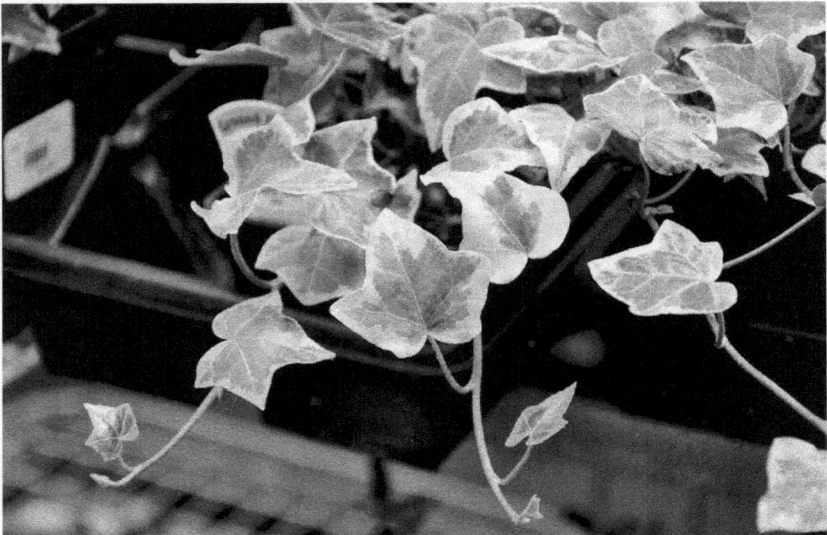

Broadleaf Lady Palm (Rhapis Excelsa)

Light: Keep in partial shade.

Temperature: Average warmth, minimum of 50 degrees in the winter.

Water: The first need is for good drainage, because all palms detest stagnant water at the roots. During the winter keep the soil slightly moist. Water more liberally in spring and summer.

Humidity: Mist leaves if room is heated. Occasionally sponge mature leaves. Avoid drafts.

Repotting: Repot only when the plant is thoroughly root-bound; as palms don't like disturbance. Compact the potting medium around the root ball.

Propagation: From seed. A temperature of 80 degrees is required, so propagation can be difficult.

Special Problems:

If you have leaves with brown tips, it's most likely caused by dry air. Mist the plant regularly during hot weather. Other causes include under-watering, cold air, and damage from touching.

If you have leaves with brown spots, it's likely leaf spot disease from over-watering or sudden chilling. Just remove the affected foliage and improve the growing conditions.

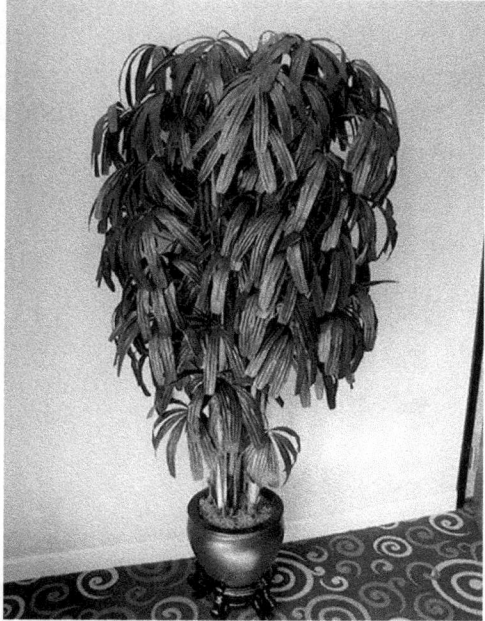

If you have yellowing leaves this is a sign of under-watering. You don't want the roots to dry out during the summer months.

If you have brown leaves and droop, this is natural for the lowest leaves. Just remove them by cutting, not by pulling. If the browning is accompanied by rotting then the problem probably is from over-watering.

If you have a cat, keep this out of reach as it is known to be toxic to cats.

Mother-in-Law's Tongue or Snake Plant (Sansevieria trifasciata or 'Laurentii')

Light: Bright light with some sun preferred, but it will also grow in shade.

Temperature: Average warmth with minimum of 50 degrees.

Water: Water moderately from spring to autumn, allowing soil to dry out slightly between waterings. In winter water every 1 – 2 months.

Avoid wetting the heart of the plant.

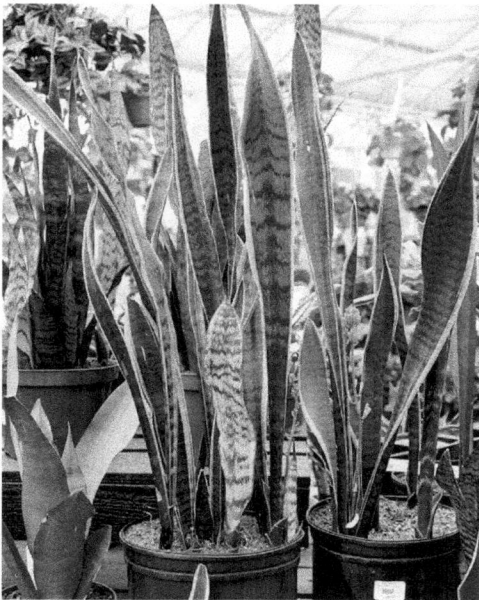

Humidity: Misting is not necessary.

Repotting: Seldom required, just repot when root-bound.

Propagation: Remove offset by cutting off at base. Allow to dry before inserting in new soil. Alternatively, divide up plant.

Special Problems: If you have leaves that are yellow and dying back, it is likely from basal rot disease. The general cause is from overwatering in the winter. If the whole of the base is affected, use the upper foliage as leaf cuttings and then discard the plant. If only part of the plant is affected, remove it from the pot and cut off the diseased section. Dust cut the surface with sulphur and repot. Keep it dry and move it to a warmer spot.

If you have rot in the base in winter and it is not overwatered, this is likely from cold damage. Sanseviera can be quickly damaged at 40 degrees or below; 50 degrees is the minimum temperature for safe winter care.

If you have brown blotches on the leaves this is likely from a non-infectious disorder that starts at the tips and works downward along the leaf. There is no known cause and no known cure.

Devils Ivy or Golden Pothos (Epiremnum oureum)
Light: Well lit but sunless spot. Variegation will fade in poor light.
Temperature: Average warmth with a minimum of 50 degrees
in winter.
Water: Water liberally from spring to autumn, but let soil dry out slightly between waterings. Water sparingly in winter.
Humidity: Mist leaves frequently.
Repotting: Repot, if necessary, in spring.
Propagation: Take stem cuttings in spring or summer; use a rooting hormone. Keep soil rather dry and then leave in dark until rooted.

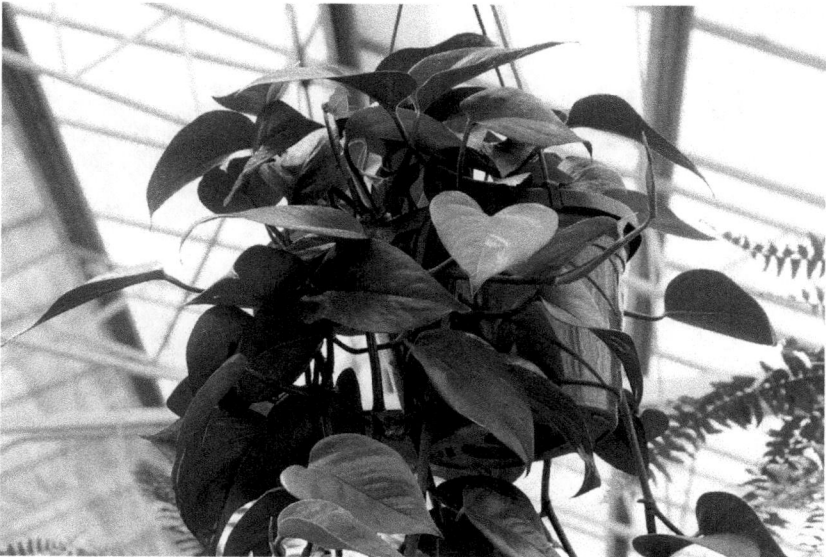

Special Problems:
If you have yellowing, falling leaves and rotting stems it's likely caused by overwatering especially in the winter.
If you have brown leaf edges and brown spots on the leaf surface tit-is likely a case of under watering during

the growing season. The soil should become dry between waterings but the root ball must not be allowed to dry out.

If you have curled limb leaves and rotting stems, this is likely caused by cold air damage. Scinapsus is extremely sensitive to a sudden drop in temperature below 50 degrees.

Heart Leaf Philodendron (Philodendron Oxycardium)

Light: Keep out of direct sunlight. Keep in light shade or moderate brightness.

Temperature: Average warmth, minimum 55 degrees in winter.

Water: During winter keep the soil just moist and make sure it is not waterlogged. For the rest of the year, water thoroughly and regularly.

Humidity: Keep the air moist in the summer and keep in a heated room in winter. Surround the plant with peat and mist the leaves.

Repotting: Transfer to a larger pot in spring every 2 – 3 years.

Propagation: Cuttings require warm conditions. In the summer, air layer the plant.

If you have a cat, keep this out of reach, as it is toxic to cats.

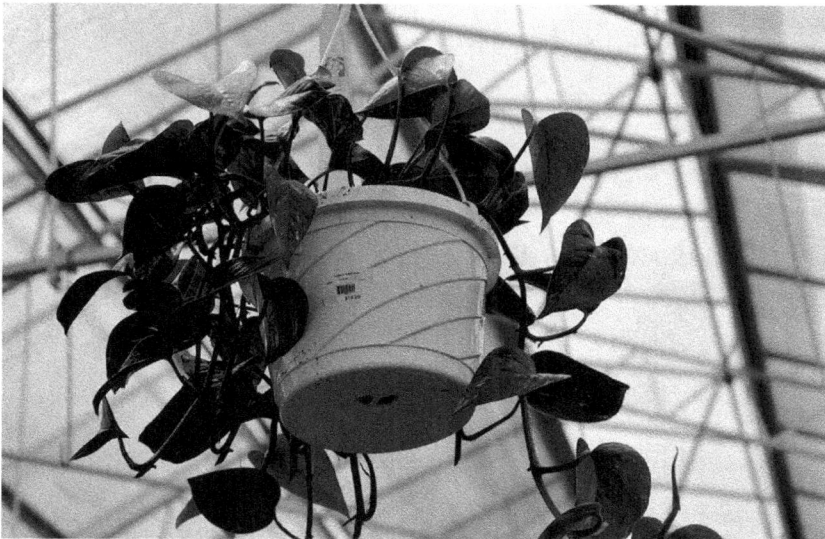

Boston Fern (Nephrolepis Exaltata "Bostoniensis")

Light: Despite popular opinion, ferns are not shade lovers indoors, as most varieties originated in the dappled brightness of tropical woodland. Good indirect light is the proper location; an east or north-facing windowsill would be ideal.

Temperature: Average warmth, cool but not cold nights are desirable. The best temperature range is 60 – 70 degrees. The minimum for most types is about 50 degrees, and ferns may suffer at more than 75 degrees.

Water: Soil must be kept moist at all times and never allowed to dry out, but this does not mean constantly soggy. Waterlogging will lead to rotting. Reduce watering in winter.

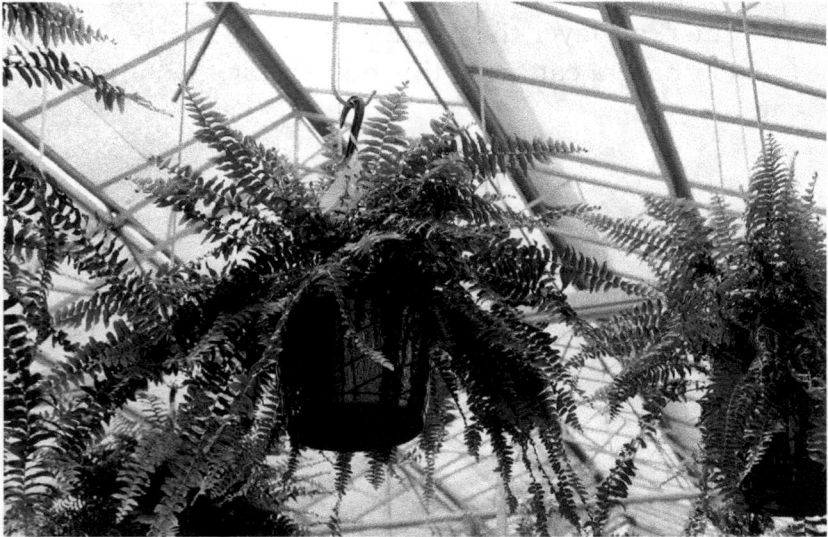

Humidity: Moist air is necessary for nearly all ferns. Mist fronds regularly.

Repotting: Repot in spring when the roots fill the pot. Most young specimens will probably require annual repotting. Do not bury the crown of the plant.

Propagation: The simplest way is to divide the plant into 2 or 3 pieces in early spring if it produces rhizomes. Some ferns produce young plants at the ends of runners and this is one of them.

Special Problems:

If you have brown dots or lines regularly arranged on the underside of fronds, these are cases of spores. This is an indication that the frond is mature and healthy. The spores produced inside these spore cases can be used for propagation.

If you have brown shells irregularly scattered on the fronds, this is a scale and insect problem.

If you have yellowing fronds beginning at the base of the plant, this is a problem with it being too warm. A common complaint with ferns is that they are set too close to radiators. Few ferns can tolerate very high temperatures. If the plant is also limp and wilting, the likely cause is incorrect watering.

Mature fronds will develop brown spots and fall.

If you have fronds that are yellowing with brown tips and there is no new growth, the problem is probably that the air is too dry.

If you have pale fronds with "scorch marks" on the surface this is probably from too much sun. Ferns must be protected from midday sunshine in the summer.

If you have pale fronds and weak growth, it's likely caused by not enough fertilizer. Ferns need feeding, little and often during the growing season.

If you have fronds that are dying back, it's probably dry air and dry soil.

Bamboo Palm (Chamaedorea Sefritzii), Weeping Fig (Fiscus Benjamina), Red-Edged Dracena (Dracaena Marginata), Peace Lily (Spathiphyllum), Bamboo Palm

(Chamaedorea Sefritzii), Spider Plant (Chlorophytum Comosum): See details under benzene-purifying plants.

Plants for Trichloroethylene:

Bamboo Palm or Reed Palm (Chamaedorea Sefritzii)
Gerbera Daisy (Gerbera Jamesonii)
Peace Lily (Spathiphyllum)
Red-Edged Dracena (Dracaena Marginata)
Warneck Dracaena (Dracaena Deremensis 'Warneckii)
Pot Mum or Florist's Chrysanthemum (Chrysanthemum Morifolium)

Plants for Xylene and Toluene:

Dumb Cane (Exotica Dieffenbachiaoestedii)
Light: Partial shade in summer but bright in winter.
Temperature: Average or above average warmth with a minimum of 60 degrees in the winter.
Water: Water regularly from spring to autumn. Water sparingly in winter.
Humidity: Mist frequently. Surround plant with damp peat. Wash leaves occasionally.
Repotting: Repot in spring every year.
Propagation: Remove and pot up the top crown of leaves using a rooting hormone, and provide bottom heat. Use two- to three-inch pieces of the stem as cane cuttings. Some varieties produce daughter plants at the base, which can be removed and used as cuttings.

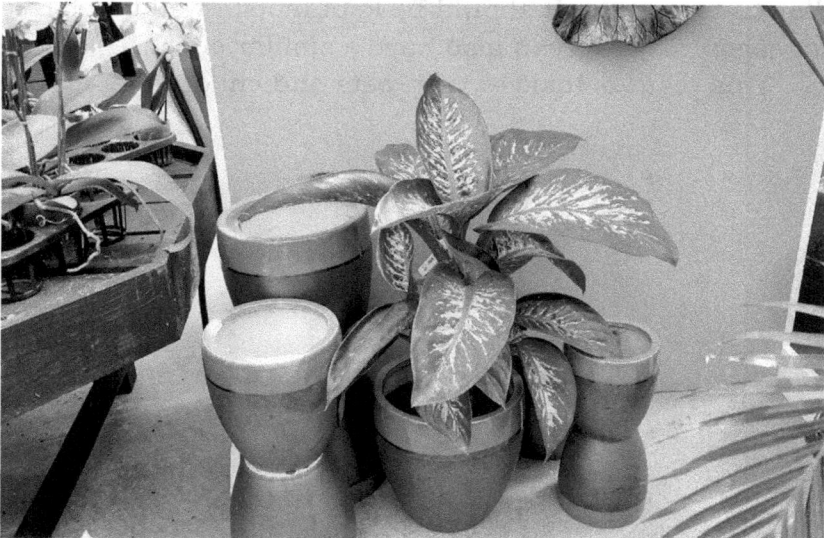

Special problems:
Watch for insects such as scale and red spider mites.

If the stem base is soft and discolored it is probably from stem rot disease. This can be caused by over-watering and low temperatures. If the damage is slight just cut out the diseased area and spray with carbendazim and repot. If the damage is severe, discard the plant and use the top as a cutting.

If the leaves have lost their color, this is probably caused by direct sunlight or excessive brightness; just move it to a shadier spot.

If there is a loss of leaves, the temperature is probably too cool. Avoid drafts on young leaves. Old leaves will drop naturally with age.

If the lower leaves are yellow and wilted, it's probably caused by low winter temperatures or cold drafts. This plant can survive 50 – 65 degrees, but the lower leaves will suffer.

If the leaves have brown edges, then the soil has been allowed to dry out. It should be kept moist at all times but not soggy. Cold air can also have a similar effect.

This plant is toxic to both pets and children.

Dendrobium Orchid (Dendrobium sp.)

Light: Provide bright light, with up to 50 percent sun, ideally in an east, west or lightly shaded south window.

Temperature: Mature plants need a 15 – 20 degree difference between night and day, ideally nighttime temperatures of 60 – 65 degrees and day temperatures of 80 – 90 degrees. Temperatures of up to 95 degrees are beneficial if humidity and air circulation are increased. Low temperatures (below 50 degrees) may cause leaf drop.

Water: Keep evenly moist while inactive during the "dormant" season. Allow to dry between waterings after growth is mature (indicated by terminal leaf).

Humidity: Dendrobiums need 50 – 60 percent humidity. Set plants on trays over moistened pebbles.

Fertilizer: Plants should be fed regularly during their active growing period. The exact fertilizer used will depend on the mix in which the plant is growing. A general rule is to use a balanced (10-10-10) fertilizer weekly or every two

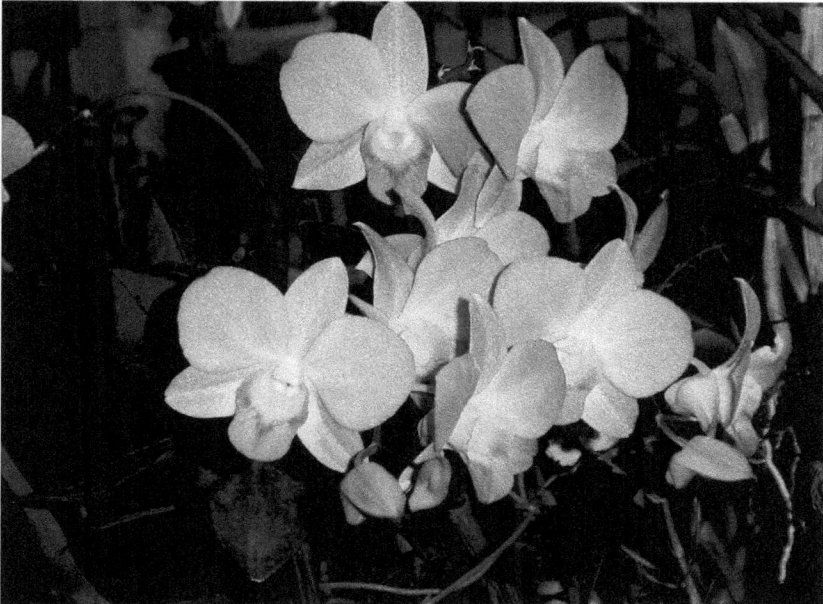

weeks at ¼ to ½ of the recommended formula.

Repotting: Should be done every two to three years before potting mix breaks down. Pot firmly in a medium pot, giving aeration and ample drainage, allowing enough room for two years' growth. Dendrobiums grow best in pots that are somewhat small for the size of the plant.

Pygmy Date Palm (Phoenix Roebelenii)

Light: Keep in partial shade.

Temperature: Average warmth, minimum of 50 degrees in the winter.

Water: The first need is for good drainage; all palms detest stagnant water at the roots. During the winter, keep the soil slightly moist. Water more liberally in spring and summer.

Humidity: Mist leaves if room is heated. Occasionally sponge mature leaves. Avoid drafts.

Repotting: Repot only when the plant is thoroughly root-bound; palms don't like disturbance. Compact the soil around the root ball.

Propagation: From seed. A temperature of 80 degrees is required, so propagation is difficult.

Special Problems:

If you have leaves with brown tips it's probably caused by dry air. Mist the plant regularly during hot

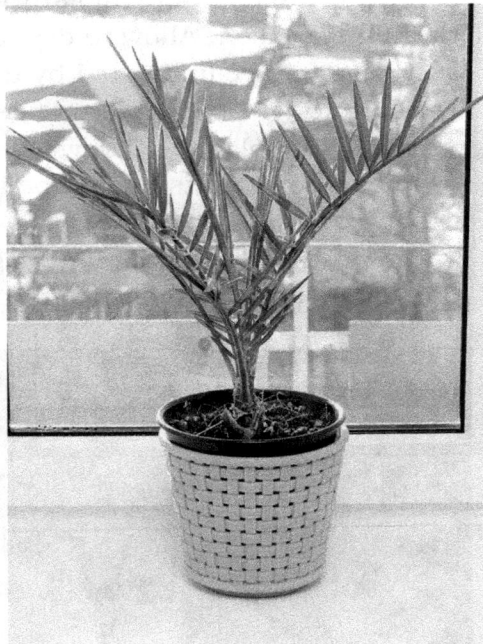

weather. Other causes include under-watering, cold air, and damage by touching.

If you have leaves with brown spots it could be leaf spot disease from over-watering or sudden chilling. Just remove the affected foliage and improve the growing conditions. Another cause i- the use of hard water.

If you have yellowing leaves this is a sign of under watering. You don't want the roots to dry out during the summer months.

If you have brown leaves and droop, this is natural for the lowest leaves. Just remove by cutting, but not pulling. If the browning is accompanied by rotting, then the problem is likely- overwatering.

Bamboo Palm or Reed Palm (Chamaedorea Sefritzii)
Boston Fern (Nephrolepis Exaltata "Bostoniensis")
Broadleaf Lady Palm (Rhapis Excelsa)
Peace Lily (Spathiphyllum 'Mauna Loa')
Red-edged Dracaena (Dracaena Marginata)
Golden Pothos
Pot Mum or Florist's Chrysanthemum

Plants for Ammonia:

Broadleaf Lady Palm (Rhapis Excelsa)
Peace lily (Spathiphyllum 'Mauna Loa')
Pot Mum or Florist's Chrysanthemum
(Chrysanthemum Morifolium)

CHAPTER 6

THE ULTIMATE DEFENSE

In Chapter 1 we saw that the greatest problem for the asthmatic is not the supposed pollutants that air purifier filters can reduce. What matters is not the micron count or whether a purifier is considered a medical device. Your nose is superior to the machine as far as filtration goes, and it is able to not only filter air but moisten and warm it to the temperature of the blood, which is something a machine is not capable of.

In Chapter 2 we have examined both dust and dust mites. The solution is fresh air flowing into your living quarters and proper nasal breathing, as well as good old-fashioned cleanliness.

In Chapter 3 we looked at how air purifiers do not purify the air but just filter it.

Finally, in Chapter 4 we noted that the sole champions in true air purification are better than air purifying systems. Furthermore, plants naturally put ozone in check, unlike some brands of air purifiers that actually add to it.

Another Perspective on Plants

Some researchers, including the EPA Indoor Air Division, remain unconvinced that houseplants are the answer to cleaning indoor air.

The reasons for their doubt include:

Houseplants should not be your sole defense against indoor air pollution. Pollution should instead be eliminated at its source, according to The Pros Who Know, by reducing the amount of synthetic material in your home or office, and by making sure buildings are well ventilated.

Your home or office building is not a controlled research lab, so you can't really determine the number of plants needed in your environment. It's common knowledge that plants process chemicals in the air, but the rates and effectiveness can't be proven outside the laboratory setting. Too many plants can actually raise your humidity levels, encouraging mold and bacteria in the building. Your indoor humidity should be between 35 and 65 percent.

Soil does breed mold, bacteria, and mildew. Be careful that you don't over-water your plants, and keep mold under control by mulching plants with an inch of fine gravel on top of the soil surface.

Plant-growing essentials:

It makes sense to reduce the amount of synthetics in your environment, but this is easier said than done. Real wood furniture or non-synthetic building materials can be expensive, and the consequences of having too many plants are insignificant compared with an excess of pollutants from a house full of synthetic materials.

Plants can be used in conjunction with other natural methods, or even with an air purifier. If you keep your windows open and allow fresh air to flow through, this will help minimize the humidity indoors. Not over-watering your plants is a good idea, but keep in mind that bacteria is vital and will thrive with or without moist soil. The bacterial by-product is what fertilizes the soil to nourish the plants in the first place. Moreover, there are always bacteria present in the air that you breathe with or without plants, and the filters of air purifiers don't eliminate them all. Just take care of your immune system and your diet, and bacteria won't be much of a bother.

After all of this, what can we do to truly make our office space or home environment the ultimate in environmental defense.

Defense with an Air Purifier

Just like in real estate, the three most important things must be addressed:
Location.
Location.
Location.

You should focus on the rooms that you and your family spend most of your time in. This will vary from individual to individual, but one thing you can be sure of is that these places are most vital:

- Bedrooms.
- Bathrooms.
- Kitchens.
- Living rooms.
- Family rooms.
- Office rooms.
- Sewing rooms.
- Play rooms.

Now for the office environment, specifically a corporate-type office:

- ☐ Break rooms.
- ☐ Lobby/waiting areas.
- ☐ Cafeteria/lounge.
- ☐ Managerial offices.
- ☐ Conference rooms.
- ☐ Work stations.

You should also consider the type of synthetics present in these areas, the size of the areas, and the number of people present in these areas (more so for the office).

How you factor these in is crucial to the effectiveness of your environmental defensive perimeter. Why? First off, it is essential to identify the type of chemicals leaking into the air in order to put the right plants in this area to help negate this. Then you must also factor in the type of lighting and atmosphere required by the plant type. Furthermore, the more people you have present and the smaller the space, the greater the impact of exposure over a longer period of time. You need to also consider the degradation of air quality from the exhalation of a larger number of people in a smaller space. You mix this in along with the toxins from synthetic materials, and you have a set-up for health issues waiting to happen. This is why in the home you will certainly need to add some green to your bathroom, because of the confinement of space, especially if there is no window. If you spend a lot of time in your garage, you will need plenty of plants, especially if you usually keep the garage door closed.

Why are plants a good addition to an environment that contains an air purifier? Plants will extend the life of the filter for an air purifier, saving you money. And with a little care, your plants will last much longer than the filters of that machine.

Plants produce oxygen, something that the machine fails to do, and plants also filter your air on the molecular level through the negative ions that they produce.

Plants can also humidify that dry indoor air that you breathe. Plants have a positive impact on reducing ozone levels.

The best plan is to put your air purifier in a central location and arrange your plants around furniture and near the places where toxins are leaking, so they can be negated at the source. The general recommendation is one 6-inch plant for every 100 square feet of living or office space. Keep in mind that this is the minimum determined through the NASA study in the 1980s.

The All-Stars

These listed plants negate benzene, formaldehyde, trichloroethylene, xylene, toluene, and ammonia:
Chrysanthemum and Peace Lily

These plants all negate benzene, along with formaldehyde, trichloroethylene, xylene, and toluene:

- ☐ Golden Pothos
- ☐ Peace Lily
- ☐ Chrysanthemum
- ☐ Red-edged Dracaena
- ☐ Warneck Dracaena (not formaldehyde)
- ☐ English Ivy (not trichloroethylene)
- ☐ Janet Craig (not trichloroethylene)

These plants all negate benzene, formaldehyde, and trichloroethylene:

- ☐ Peace Lily
- ☐ Golden Pothos
- ☐ Chrysanthemum
- ☐ Red-edged Dracaena
- ☐ Snake Plant
- ☐ English Ivy (not trichloroethylene)
- ☐ Janet Craig (not trichloroethylene)

In the set-up of a defensive perimeter with air purifiers (aside from the use of plants), there are four other powerful components: beeswax candles, charcoal briquettes, activated charcoal, and Himalayan Crystal Salt Lamps. Try to think of things in the terms of a 360-degree military perimeter, in which you establish interlinking fire. How is this so? It is because you have an overlap of protection, such as the elimination of positive ions through the plants, beeswax candles, Himalayan Crystal Salt Lamps, and the fresh air from open windows. Remember that these same negative ions are filtering your air on a molecular level, and rather than removing the airborne pollutants, it neutralizes them by binding them tight long enough for you to clean them up with a healthy dose of daily upkeep.

Beeswax Candles and Salt Lamps

These can be wonderful additions to your home environmental defense. Particles such as dust, dirt, and pollutants in the air carry a positive charge; that's why they are suspended in the air. But negative ions from burning beeswax can negate the positive charge of contaminants. Here's what you need to know about beeswax candles.

The term "pure" on a label means just 51 percent of an ingredient. Many supplies sell

"pure" beeswax candles with a combination of 51 percent beeswax and 49 percent paraffin. Look for a label that says 100% pure beeswax – these candles are orange in color and smell like honey. Best locations for these are in between plants in the room.

These lamps produce negative ions and can be quite soothing. The pinkish, orange, reddish hues from the lamp create a naturally relaxing atmosphere. Salt crystals can vary back and forth between a crystal state and a liquid state. With a little heat provided by the bulb and changing the surface temperature of the crystal, water molecules are attracted from the cooler surrounding air and condensing on the surface of the lamp. This causes a split of the positive sodium and negative chloride ions. The negative chloride ions help bind to those positively charged pollutants in the air. These lamps also help dehumidify the air if you have an overabundance of plants.

If there is too much condensation where it appears that the lamp is sweating, this may be an indication that the surrounding environment is too moist for it to function properly. If this happens, just move the lamp to a different location.

Also be wary of the following:

- ☐ Dipping your lamp in water.
- ☐ Exposing it to rain.
- ☐ Exposing it to environments with heavy moisture.

☐ Basements with lack of ventilation and high humidity.

☐ Washing your lamp with water – wash it down with a damp cloth instead.

It is a good idea to store it in a plastic bag to keep it from pooling water if it is not being actively used, and avoid placing it directly on top of electronic devices. Here are some tips to figure out the right size of lamp or lamps to provide you with the best coverage:

☐ In a room of about 216 square feet a lamp weighing between 5 and 7 lbs.

☐ In a room of about 323 square feet a lamp weighing 7 – 9 lbs.

☐ In a room of about 474 square feet a lamp weighing 10 – 12 lbs.

☐ In a room of about 753 square feet a lamp weighing 15 – 20 lbs.

You can achieve the right weight by square footage by mixing several small to large lamps. It does not have to be exact, just close to that weight amount, and even better to add some beeswax candles and some plants.

Briquettes and Activated Charcoal

Aside from helping with a barbecue, these little wonders can aid you in many other ways. One good use of charcoal is to eliminate excess humidity. Just put some briquettes in a tin or an empty can, punch a few holes in the lid, and set it in a humid area. You should replace the charcoal every few months. You can place these inconspicuously around some of your plants to reduce raised humidity levels. To reduce odors, use activated charcoal instead of charcoal briquettes.

Activated charcoal is specially treated to increase its surface area to adsorb chemicals, even if there is no ventilation or air been forced along its surface.

You can purchase granulated active charcoal and put it in "breathable" sachets. Set or hang them in areas likely to be emitting toxic gases.

Purchase an activated charcoal/carbon filter and place it in an area where it would be most effective.

A source for good quality activated charcoal is here: buyactivatedcharcoal.com/product/pure_non-scents/odor_control

Q: What is the best method to eliminate gaseous chemicals from indoor air?

A: Ventilation, activated carbon in the form of granules in sachets, use of activated carbon filters, and plants that remove gases from your environment.

Other Measures

These measures are crucial with or without an air purifier. For the ultimate in home or office environmental defense, include the following:

A major reduction or elimination of the use of synthetic candles in exchange for soy and beeswax candles.

A major reduction or elimination of conventional aerosol type sprays in exchange for more organic-based methods of air freshening.

A major reduction or elimination of chemical-laden cleaning products in exchange for more organic-based products.

Give your ultimate air filtration system (your nose) the TLC it deserves by breathing through it and fulfilling its intended purpose.

Open up the windows in your home and allow the breeze to purify your air. (This may not be possible at the office, but if possible, do it.)

Active ventilation systems will be aided greatly by the addition of plants and other measures in this book.

Q: What if I live in an area where the outdoor air is heavily polluted?

A: Depending on the type of pollution and how high it is – such as from nearby factories – it's helpful to open the windows and ventilate for short durations off and on. It's also highly advisable to have an abundance of plants inside, perhaps with a dehumidifier to keep extra moisture in check if the windows are always or often kept shut.

Why *Not* to Buy an Air Purifier

You should consider that the following points are *not* good reasons for purchasing an air purifier:

- ☐ It filters a proportionate amount of air.
- ☐ It removes pollutants such as dust, pollen, mold spores, odors, and dust mites.
- ☐ It has a great filter that is able to further trap bacteria and other airborne particles.
- ☐ It is doctor-recommended.
- ☐ It is touted as a medical class device.
- ☐ It has the lowest micron reduction rate.

These are obviously the premium selling points used to get you to part with your money. In other words, I would not advise you to go out and purchase an air purifier for any of the reasons that are typically used to persuade you to make the purchase. Yes, air purifiers do a wonderful job at *neutralizing the pollutants in the air*, but they fail to live up to the name air purifier – air filter is more appropriate.There is no good reason to spend money on an air purifier to purify your air, because it is not designed to do that and it can't fulfill this task. However, if you want to *filter* your air, then one of these systems will suffice (in conjunction with the other measures in this book) to build your ultimate environmental defense.

Sources and More Information

Adam J. (1913) Asthma and Its Radical Treatment London, England: The Riverside Press Limited

Betül Ayşe Sin (2012). The Impact of Allergic Rhinitis on Asthma: Current View, Allergic Rhinitis, www..intechopen.com/download/get/type/pdfs/id/32964

California Environmental Protection Agency (2006) Beware of Ozone-generating Indoor "Air Purifiers" www.arb.ca.gov/research/indoor/ozone_gen_fact_sheet-a.pdf

Collier Engineer Co. (1899) A Treatise On Architecture And Building Construction Vol 4: Plumbing And Gas-Fitting, Heating And Ventilation, Painting And Decorating, Estimating And Calculating Quantities New York: Press of Eaton & Maines

DeNoon J. D. (2006) Ozone Generators Create Home Smog Air Purifiers That Produce Ozone May Be Hurting Your Health webmd.com/news/20060511/ozone-generators-home-smog?page=2

Kairaitis, K., Garlick, S. R., Wheatley, J. R., & Amis, T. C. (1999). Route of breathing in patients with asthma. Chest,116(6), 1646-52. search.proquest.com/ docview/200478711?accountid=158302

Lauren (2012, 8 September) Beeswax Candles and Allergies: An Effective Solution, empowered sustenance.com/beeswax-candles-and-allergies-an-effective-solution/

Ministry of Education (2007) Designing Quality Learning Spaces: Ventilation & Indoor Quality Air www.minedu.govt.nz

Pros Who Know (2010, 01, March) Best Houseplants to Improve Indoor Air Quality proswhoknow.wordpress.com/2010/03/01/best-houseplants-to-Improve-indoor-air-quality/

Readers Digest (n.d.) 5 Things To Do with Charcoal Briquettes www.readersdigest.ca/home-garden/5-things/5-things-do-charcoal-briquettes

Rixon D. (2010, 12 February) Unusual Uses: Charcoal
www.diylife.com/2010/02/12/unusual-uses-charcoal/
Robins Y.E. (1860) Ventilation as Influencing Health and
Longevity. nytimes.com/1860/03/23/news/ventilation-as-
influencing-health-and-longevity-lecture-by-mr-ey-robbins.html
Yeager J. (2010, 22 December) 10 Handy Alternative Uses of
Charcoal thedailygreen.com/living-
green/blogs/savemoney/uses-of-charcoal
Science Daily (September 9, 2009) Houseplants Cut Indoor
Ozone sciencedaily.com/releases/2009/09/090908103634.htm

ABOUT THE
AUTHOR

JULIAN COX is an AADP Certified Health Coach with a diploma in Colour Therapy. He graduated with high honors from the American Intercontinental University in 2010 obtaining a B.A. in Human Resource Management, and has studied to become a Health Coach at the Institute for Integrative Nutrition in 2012. He received a diploma in Colour Therapy from the School of Natural Health Sciences in 2012.

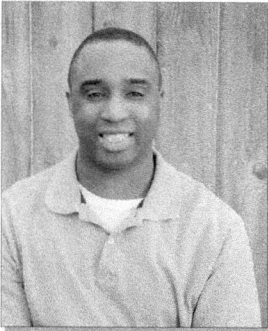

Due to a neurological injury he received while serving with the United States Army in 2006 during a final deployment to Iraq, he has become passionate about health. He has spent years turning his own chronic condition around without the use of drugs, and is on a mission to help others achieve some of the great successes that he has.

In the process of his journey of continued recovery, Julian Cox has learned many fundamental aspects that seem to be overlooked in the industry of health and wellness. Therefore it has become his passion to help people realize that great health can be achieved at a fraction of what many assume. Best wishes – and to your health!

www.ingramcontent.com/pod-product-compliance
Lightning Source LLC
Chambersburg PA
CBHW052055270326
41931CB00012B/2770